D0307769

OF01032

Books should be returned to the SDH Library on or before
the date stamped above unless a renewal has been arranged

Salisbury District Hospital Library

Telephone: Salisbury (01722) 336262 extn. 4432 / 33

Out of hours answer machine in operation

Dedicated to our daughters
and to their daughters
and
to Mat, Bo and Tom,
the births of whom
transformed my life

Midwifery Teams and Caseloads

Caroline Flint SRN, SCM, ADM

Illustrated by
Helen Chown BA(Hons) Fine Art

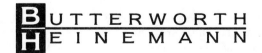

BUTTERWORTH
HEINEMANN

Butterworth-Heinemann Ltd
Linacre House, Jordan Hill, Oxford OX2 8DP

℟ A member of the Reed Elsevier Group

OXFORD   LONDON   BOSTON
MUNICH   NEW DELHI   SINGAPORE   SYDNEY
TOKYO   TORONTO   WELLINGTON

First published 1993
Reprinted 1994

British Library Cataloguing in Publication Data
Flint, Caroline
    Midwifery Teams and Caseloads
    I. Title
    618.2

ISBN 0 7506 0987 7

Typeset by TecSet Ltd, Wallington, Surrey
Printed and bound in Great Britain by
Biddles Ltd, Guildford and King's Lynn

Contents

Preface

This is an essentially practical book to help midwives to provide the continuity of care that women have been asking for. The book addresses the difficulties of achieving change and gives practical and achievable targets for achieving this change.

Duty rosters from many different Team Schemes are included, and the reader can choose the type of scheme that would best suit her and her Unit. Ways to enable a Team to grow and gel together are suggested, as are workshops to enable Groups and Teams to learn about each other and to work together happily. Health Care Assistants, staffing a GP Unit and Birth Centre and a description of Independent Midwives working in partnership – midwives having their own caseloads – are discussed and explored.

This is a book which could transform the care of women in the United Kingdom – every suggestion and discussion is well researched and is in line with the principles behind the latest Select Committee Report.

Acknowledgements

So many people have helped in the production of this book it is hard to know where to start. As he has for the past 29 years, Giles Flint, my beloved husband, has been a tower of strength and encouragement, Janet Andrews has worked hard by typing, collecting and 'phoning to enable this book to be written, Val Taylor my midwifery partner has given me a great deal of encouragement.

Information has been generously given by Jean Keats, Pauline Wells, Margaret Stockwell, Valerie Outram, Heather Bower, Helen Minns, Jean Cushing and many others. Thanks are due to the staff at MIDIRS (the Midwives Information and Resource Service) who have as usual answered my queries and requests with efficiency and enthusiasm. Thanks are also due to Jan Ayres and Judith Ions at the Royal College of Midwives' Library for help generously given.

To Suzanne Truttero and the midwifery managers in Riverside Health Authority grateful thanks are due for a unique opportunity to work as a Consultant in the management of change, and further thanks are due to the midwifery staff in that Health Authority.

The thoughts and ideas expressed in this book have been collected over the years – there are dozens of people who should be acknowledged for feeding me with ideas and visions over those years, if your name isn't mentioned here please forgive me. If I wrote all the names of those who have helped me over the time I have been researching for this book, the subsequent document would be almost as big as the finished book, all I can say is thank you to all those midwives and women who have been so generous to me.

1
Introduction

Women have been asking for continuity of carer for as long as any of us can remember. In some Units genuine attempts have been made to provide some women with a midwife to attend them throughout their labour with whom they have been able to form a relationship during their pregnancy. But in many Units the changes have merely been cosmetic.

Frequently, changing to a 'Team Scheme' means that women are allocated to a specific team of midwives, but that Team can be anything up to 25 members which, as far as the woman is concerned, is totally meaningless. By looking at a woman's notes in the postnatal period it is quite simple to see how many different care-givers a woman sees in your Unit, by counting how many signatures there are throughout the pregnancy, labour and postnatal period and by being aware that this probably represents between one-third and one-half of the health care professionals who have actually dealt with the woman.

The postnatal ward clerk does not write in the woman's notes, nor does a nursery nurse, nor someone who just gives her a little bit of breastfeeding advice, nor does the person who tests her urine in the antenatal clinic, nor the phlebotomist who takes her blood on at least three occasions in her pregnancy. One needs to be aware of how many hidden people there are when going through a woman's notes.

In this book I am exploring different ways of providing continuity of carer, some better and some less effective than others. We shall be looking at midwife teams and at midwives with individual caseloads and working together with other midwives to form a Group Practice, we shall look at Teams based in hospital and those based wherever the women need them. We shall look at the costs of providing continuity of care and the benefits and disadvantages both for the women and for the midwives.

We are going to look at the enjoyment and job satisfaction that continuity of carer provides for midwives but we shall also explore those situations that cause them stress and the ways different midwives find to deal with stress and anxiety. Continuity of care given by midwives also affects other health professionals – we shall explore the effect on GPs and obstetricians and other health professionals that we work with. Finally we need to explore the implications for midwifery managers, women and their families, and of course the midwives themselves.

Change is extraordinarily difficult and painful, but from the Report of the House of Commons Select Committee which published its report in 1992 (the Winterton Report) it is quite obvious, from the huge volume of evidence from women, that they are no longer satisfied with us telling them that continuity of carer is too idealistic or too costly or too difficult to provide, this is what women are demanding of us – we cannot resist their pressure any longer. The service we produce is for them and we must make it receptive to their needs and demands. We HAVE to provide them with systems that enable them to get to know their midwife.

What women are asking for is only reasonable; at one of the most intimate times in her entire life a woman is asking for someone to be with her who she knows and trusts, someone she has been able to build a relationship with. We are human beings and continuity is extremely important to us. I always wait until the days my own dentist is at the dental surgery, I am rarely willing to see his (I'm sure equally competent) partner. It's the same with my car – Fred sees to my cars, every time, and if Fred says that the big end has gone I know that he is right, and I also know that Fred will fix it as well as he is able and at as reasonable a price as possible because, after all the years we have been together, I trust Fred.

For the house it's Phil. Phil always paints the house, or clears the drains, or mends the garage door. I'd never dream of asking a stranger to deal with my S bend – even less would I think of asking a stranger to help me at my time of greatest vulnerability, when giving birth.

Humans are mammals, all mammals only have a few of their fellows with them during labour and birth and those fellows are trusted and known whether the mammal is a dolphin, a pet cat or a deer. Surely, human mammals should be respected in the same way as we respect our pet dog or cat. We would never entrust them to someone they didn't know when they are in labour – we care for them too much. What does it say about our usual treatment of labouring women that we can abandon them just when they need us most? We have to change, we have to explore together how we can change the way we work.

Throughout this book I shall be trying to ensure that you are looking at the care women are receiving with your eyes and senses centred on the central core – that for women continuity of carer means having someone with her in labour with whom she has been able to form a relationship during her pregnancy.

Quite a large body of research has been amassed on continuity of carer and we need to look at and evaluate everything that we can gain access to. Many of the studies contain quite small numbers of women but there are two studies which contain a large number of women – the Know Your Midwife research carried out between 1983 and 1985 at St George's Hospital in Tooting which looked at 1001 women, and the research done by Anne Oakley, Lynda Rajan and Adrian Grant between 1986 and 1987 which looked at 509 women (Oakley *et al.*, 1990).

Midwives who provide care for a woman all the way through her pregnancy, labour and the puerperium often feel that working this way increases the learning opportunities for that midwife. She sees all the facets of a continuum and she is able to observe the outcome of her practice and her clinical decisions, so that if her suturing was not as good as it should have been she will see the perineum breaking down, or if she made a recommendation that the woman declined to take, she can see that the woman was right or that it would have been better for her to have taken the midwife's advice.

Many midwives involved in continuity of carer appreciate the support they have from the women they are becoming involved with. A close friendship is formed between the mother and the midwife and this enables the midwife to be braver and enables the mother to be more powerful. Although this effect of continuity of carer has never been evaluated (probably because it is almost impossible to do so), it would appear that women are empowered by the relationship they have with 'their' midwife, and that they feel the effects of having 'a friend on the inside'; these benefits also happen to the midwife who feels appreciated, and more powerful on behalf of 'her' client.

When midwives work together in a group practice or team, if they work hard at building a good team spirit they will find enormous support from each other and professional development from their conversations with each other. They will also find a bond of deep affection – love will flow between the members of their group which will sustain them when life is hard or all the babies come at once and they are exhausted.

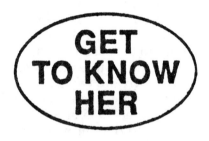

Jean Ball, in her treatise 'Birthrate', describes women who she has named Category X (Ball, 1992). These are women who go into a Labour Ward and who are subsequently discovered to not be in established labour; they are either sent home or admitted to an antenatal ward to await events. Jean Ball points out that the admission of these women is extremely expensive for the National Health Service (NHS). In the seven Maternity Units that she surveyed she estimates cost savings of between £2000 and £14 000 per month if these admissions were reduced by a half.

Women admitted as Category X take up midwifery and medical time on the labour ward, they take up beds and they take up the use of equipment and are subject to greater intervention, because although some of them are sent home a great many are kept in the hospital to await the start of labour or to have labour induced. Jean Ball concludes: "If some of these savings (reducing the admissions of Category X patients) were used to fund increased community oversight of these cases then further improvements in the effectiveness and appropriateness of care could be achieved".

A study by Klein *et al.* published in 1983 showed the benefits which occur when women in early labour are assessed at home (Klein *et al.*, 1983a,b).

The study describes the data collected from 1436 low-risk women following their care during childbirth. The women lived in Oxford. Some of them had shared care with their GP, which meant that they went to their GP's surgery for antenatal care either from the Community Midwife or their GP, when they went into labour they were admitted to the John Radcliffe hospital in Oxford – they had occasional visits to the hospital for antenatal checks.

The other women had General Practitioner Unit (GP Unit) care. In the same way as the shared care group they went to their GP's surgery for antenatal care either from the Community Midwife or their GP, when they went into labour they were admitted to the John Radcliffe hospital in Oxford – they had occasional visits to the hospital for antenatal checks.

There was, however, a difference in treatment for this group which was to prove highly significant – the women in the GP Unit's group were delivered by the midwife from the GP's surgery and in the process of that, they had their labour assessed at home or, sometimes, at the GP's surgery.

The GP Unit at the John Radcliffe Hospital does not exist in a physical form. The room the Community Midwife uses is just one of the rooms in the Labour Ward, today it might be room 3, tomorrow room 9. The only real difference in the women having GP Unit care is that when the women go into labour they contact their Community Midwife and she assesses their labour at home; when the women having shared care go into labour they contact the hospital labour ward.

What was the difference in outcome for those women who had GP Unit care (that is, those women who were assessed in early labour at home by a midwife who they knew)? Here is the summary from the *British Journal of Obstetrics and Gynaecology* from February 1983 (Klein *et al.*, 1983a)

A random sample of low-risk women were equally divided into four groups of 63 nulliparae and multiparae each booked for care in an integrated general practice unit (GPU) and a shared-care (consultant) system. Selection criteria included only women who were admitted because they were in spontaneous labour or thought they were. Nulliparous women booked for shared-care came into hospital at a less advanced state of cervical dilation than those booked for the GPU and spent longer (11 compared with 8 h) in hospital before delivery; the comparable durations in multiparae were 6 and 4 h. Both the first and second stage of labour were longer in the GPU-booked women but they received less pethidine and fewer had epidural analgesia; they received less electronic fetal monitoring, augmentation and forceps delivery, and fetal distress was diagnosed less often. The 1-min Apgar score was <6 in 17.5% of infants of nulliparae booked for the shared-care system compared with 1.6% of those booked for the GPU. The intubation rate of infants of nulliparae was 11% in the shared-care system compared with no intubations in the GPU. These comparisons demonstrate the simplicity and safety of delivery of low-risk women in the GPU as compared with deliveries of similar women in a shared-care (consultant) unit.

Just by being assessed at home during early labour the system eliminated 'Category X', but it also meant that women received less analgesia, less fetal monitoring, augmentation and instrumental delivery. Their babies came out with higher Apgar scores and with less need for intubation – benefits which are cost effective for the NHS, less traumatic for the mothers and babies, and probably more empowering for the women. All this was achieved by one small intervention – the woman being assessed at home by a midwife that she knew.

What other benefits for women can we expect when all women are cared for in this way?

In the 'Know Your Midwife' scheme at St George's Hospital, Tooting, a team of four midwives looked after 250 women a year from 1983 until 1985, the benefits which accrued to the women as a result of continuity of carers were many:

1. Less analgesia in labour.
2. Feeling of 'being in control'.
3. Finding it easier to be a mother.
4. Less interventions during labour.
5. More able to take up a comfortable position in labour.
6. Less episiotomies.
7. Less antenatal admissions.

8. Cheaper antenatal consultations.
9. Greater enjoyment of antenatal care.
10. More normal deliveries.
11. Greater enjoyment of postnatal care.

The other apparent benefit following care by midwives the women were enabled to know was the 'power' factor mentioned earlier – this was never evaluated and has only been observed, never scientifically seen. Women who took part in the Know Your Midwife Scheme were more 'bolshie' than most women; something happened to them during their care and they became more assertive than they had been before and more assertive than the Control Group.

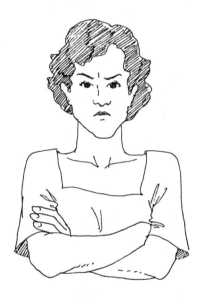

Sometimes they would refuse to have a medical student with them during labour, sometimes they would decide not to take the advice given to them by the midwife or doctor. Sometimes they would complain about the food – either the quality or the quantity. We were never conscious that they complained about us – the midwives – in fact they were extremely loyal and supportive to us, but they were just more confident of their own rights and of how things should be, and they felt that they had a right to express their feelings, probably because during their pregnancy they had experienced care from midwives who expected them to have ideas and preferences of their own.

For instance, in the St George's notes there was a space for women to write down their Birth Plan. About 18 months into the Scheme, I was seeing a woman in the Antenatal Clinic and I noticed that her Birth Plan had not been completed and I asked her what she would like to write in her Birth Plan. She said "It's up to you really, you're the expert". I felt shocked, I suddenly realised that I hadn't experienced this type of passive behaviour since the inception of the Scheme. "I can't take that sort of responsibility" I gasped, "It's your pregnancy, your labour, your baby, we need to know what you want from us at the time, we can't decide for you". This woman sticks out and remains with me even after all this time. It was because it was so uncharacteristic for the women we were dealing with not to have definite opinions and desires. These women were part of a randomised group, from a poor part of London, the mix of social classes was great, we were not dealing with specifically assertive middle class women, many of our women were quite poor, coming from very modest (sometimes extremely poor) homes.

The benefits to women are more apparent than the benefits to midwives but there are definite benefits for midwives. Let us look at the way most midwives work at present. They frequently work in hospital where they have different shifts, either 7.30 a.m. – 4.30 p.m., 12.30 p.m. – 9.30 p.m. or a night shift.

Many midwives don't know their off-duty very far in advance, sometimes they have barely a week's notice of their shifts. Relationships within the hospital are often quite strained. Many midwives have a 'best friend' or two but they feel unable to confide in any other midwives. It is impossible for a midwife to ask a more senior midwife about a mistake she thinks she might have made because the midwife knows that she will be castigated, or gossiped about or even disciplined. Time and time again midwives are asked to write a statement – just to 'cover' themselves, or the hospital, or the health authority, or the doctor – who are they 'covering' themselves against? Who is the enemy who will litigate against them? The patient – who else?

Midwives who provide continuity usually feel able to trust the women they care for, precisely because they become friends, they know each other, the midwife supports the mother, but equally the mother supports the midwife. They do not see each other as potential litigants, on different sides of the court room, they care about each other, they feel affection for each other. If anything tragic happens to the baby the parents are devastated, but so is the midwife.

I remember a very experienced midwife saying after she had delivered the stillborn son of parents she had provided continuity of care to throughout the pregnancy: "Caroline I have never felt so dreadful as this about a stillborn baby, I've delivered quite a few over the years but I've never cried about them before, I've never had vivid dreams about them before, I don't know why I can't snap out of it this time." My reply was: "You have never known the parents in this way before, you've never established such a warm and loving relationship with the parents before, you were expecting that baby too, you have had a loss too, of course you are grieving for the baby, you need to talk with and grieve with the parents." We hugged each other and had a good cry, a tragedy had occurred and she had been involved in it, it is still a tragedy even if we pretend that everything must go on as usual.

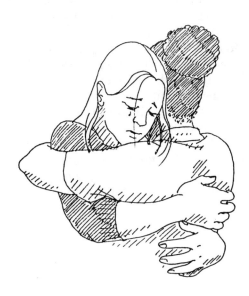

The benefits of continuity of carer are a far greater joy and involvement when things are going well, but also a far greater sadness when things don't turn out well. This is only right. When a baby dies it is a tragedy, we shouldn't just be able to take it in our stride and carry on as if nothing has happened – something has happened, a terrible tragedy has taken place, we need to acknowledge that.

She kept in touch with the parents and 2 years later delivered their fine healthy daughter. They just couldn't have anyone else with them, they had to have their dear friend who had gone through such tragedy and sadness with them – such rejoicing, it was delightful!

Not only do we need to look at all the research evaluating continuity of carer, it is also important to look at initiating change – perhaps the hardest task of all. Change is so painful and so difficult that it is worth considering whether it is really worth doing. My hypothesis is that if it does not enable women to be delivered by a midwife they have been able to get to know, is it really worth going through the agony of change to achieve something which is merely cosmetic?

We know what women want – they have been telling us for long enough and the evidence is so vast and shows up with not only every national survey into pregnant women's requests but also with every local survey. Women want the same health professional to provide them with their care throughout pregnancy, labour, delivery and the puerperium, so that they can get to know and develop a relationship with that health care professional. It is obvious that women will accept two midwives working in a partnership, but how many is too many? Can they cope with six? or ten? or only three? How many people can one make a real relationship with? This we do not know yet, but if we are setting up Teams and they consist of seven or 20 or 14, should we really be bothering? Are we deceiving ourselves that we have made improvements? Are we playing confidence tricks on women again, just as we did with domino deliveries?

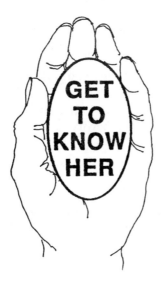

1978
Micklethwaite, Beard and Shaw
She would like, if it were possible, to have someone around during her labour who had given her some antenatal care.

1980
Short Report
I think this is what women complain about most: they do not have continuity of care which they want very much during their antenatal visits but certainly during labour and delivery.

We recognise the difficulties of providing continuity of care throughout pregnancy and labour but consider that a measure of it can be attained by better organisation.

1981
Kitzinger
there is an almost complete absence of continuity of care and each time she attends a woman sees different, anonymous faces.

1982
Maternity Services Advisory Committee
Continuity of care. It is important that the woman should be able to build up a relationship of trust with the staff she meets, and efforts should be made to involve the same group of staff at each visit.

1982
Boyd and Sellers
I was more relaxed because my midwife was with me. p. 145

By and large it is the midwife who makes or breaks a happy delivery. p. 123

These women enjoyed labour – they were given choice, they were attended by midwives they liked. p. 91

My labour was a truly delightful experience – – – attended by professional people that I regarded as friends. p. 87

1982
Royal College of Obstetricians and Gynaecologists
It has been suggested to us that women should have the same midwife to attend them in labour as in the antenatal period. We consider this continuity of care to be an ideal aim and it may be possible in some circumstances.

1983
Ong, Family Service Units
Plan effective continuity of care – women should have the opportunity of building up a relationship with one doctor, one midwife.

1983
Parents (7500 replies)
Mothers would like antenatal, delivery and postnatal care to be provided, as far as possible, by the same people. Again and again, letters expressed the anxiety that arises when seeing a different doctor at each visit to the antenatal clinic, and at being delivered by total strangers – sometimes two different shifts of total strangers if a woman had a long labour.

1986
Parents (9000 replies)
Good communications between parents and the medical staff were helped where women saw the same doctor and midwife regularly. – – – – most mothers saw different people at almost every antenatal visit and were delivered by total strangers. While full of praise for the care they received, many women wished they could have had more continuity of care through pregnancy and beyond.

1986
Association of Radical Midwives
The basic principles from which this proposal evolves are:
— That the relationship between mother and midwife is funda-
mental to good midwifery care.
— That the mother is the central person in the process of care.
— Informed choice in childbirth for women.
— Continuity of care for all childbearing women.

1987
Flint and Poulengeris
I feel that everybody would benefit from knowing the midwife
who delivers them. I found this to be extremely important when
in labour, I would have been much more nervous and scared if I
hadn't known and trusted my midwife.

It would be nice if you could see the same midwife all through
your pregnancy then during labour.

The same midwife should follow the patient from clinic to
delivery to postnatal ward and hopefully to her home afterwards.

1989
Chalmers, Enkin and Keirse
The midwife is ideally qualified to provide continuity of care, as
she is the only health professional whose training relates specifically to both the clinical and the advisory aspects of pregnancy,
labour, and the puerperium.

1991
Melia, Morgan, Wolfe and Swan
Seventy-seven per cent of women attached some importance to
continuity of midwifery care during the antenatal and postnatal
periods, and 80 per cent to knowing the delivering midwife.

The importance attached to continuity of midwifery care is
similar to previous findings. More than 65 per cent of women
gave some importance to knowing the midwife who delivers
their baby, yet in a recent survey (Which? Consumers Association) 90 per cent of women were delivered by unfamiliar hospital
staff.

1991
The Royal College of Midwives
It is important that care is arranged so that it can be provided on

a one-to-one basis by professionals able to provide continuity and consistency.

Research has shown that continuity of care from known professionals is an important factor in achieving a successful outcome to birth. Women users of the service have also specifically requested continuity of care and carer.

1992
Winterton Report
Continuity should mean the mother knows the midwife who will do the delivery. For both the hospital and home birth I saw one midwife for all antenatal check-ups, but she did not do the delivery. This is a form of continuity but it is not very useful.

A stranger meets you when you are under pressure in labour. You need to have the chance to become relaxed with and build up confidence in your birth attendant when you are not under pressure. It would be far better to see several midwives for your antenatal care, one of whom would do the delivery.

Continuity of care through pregnancy, birth and the postnatal period is of primary importance to mothers.

Women are particularly concerned about who will be with them during labour, a time when they are at their most powerless because they cannot get up and walk away if they are unhappy with what is offered. The care and attendance of a known individual at this time is of itself supportive.

We should move as rapidly as possible towards a situation in which midwives have their own caseload and take full responsibility for the women under their care.

Schemes should be set up enabling women to get to know one or two health professionals during pregnancy who will be with them during labour and delivery, whether at home or in hospital, and who will continue the care of mother and baby after birth.

We conclude that there is a strong desire among women for the provision of continuity of care and carer throughout pregnancy and childbirth, and that the majority of them regard midwives as the group best placed and equipped to provide this.

I hope this book will help you towards providing women with what they have been asking us for — good luck in your struggles to achieve this.

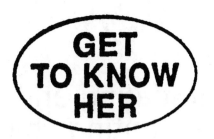

2

Initiating and implementing change

Effecting change

To effect change, especially in a large institution, is probably one of the most difficult tasks in the world. Not only is it extremely difficult, it is also extremely painful and uncomfortable for those going through it. Change upsets and distresses human beings to the very fibre and central core of their soul. Change is painful even if it is longed for and exciting. Change is painful even if the preparation has been long and deep. Change is painful even when those involved in it have been looking forward to its initiation for many years.

If change is so painful, is it worth doing? I would suggest that it really isn't worth doing unless the results will achieve real significance. The more I explore team midwifery and midwifery teams that have been set up in different hospitals and venues, the more I realise that in many places this has been change for the sake of change and that the change is a cosmetic one only.

In many of the Team Schemes set up over the past few years the fundamental issues have not been touched. There has been no fundamental change in the way women are looked after or in those people who hold the power over them and their bodies. Women have been asking for the opportunity to make a relationship with a midwife during pregnancy who is the same midwife who will look after them in labour and who delivers their baby. If the changes contemplated in your Unit, or in your Community, do not achieve that single and most important objective then the amount of effort that you and the midwives working on the ground will have to expend is probably just not worth it. If change does not achieve the end which women have been asking us for, then it is not worth doing.

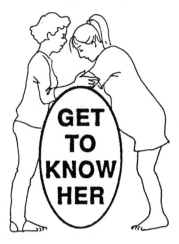

Changing someone's practice cannot be imposed from outside – it needs to come from within that person's own mind. The person needs to see the need for change and indeed they need to want to change before they can change. The problem is how do you help people to want to change? How do you steer people to throw away mores which they have held dear for years and which they have never questioned?

When we work in hospital we rarely see the effect our care is having on the people we are providing care for. We work as hard as we can and we work as well as we can. Women in general, and midwives in particular, work very hard and are extremely committed. Midwives presume that women are appreciating the amount of devotion that each individual midwife is putting in to their care. Midwives often don't realise that to the woman they are just another face – one of dozens, pleasant, kindly, but just another one.

Ways to enable people to see how it really is

In order to effect change it is necessary to help the midwife to see what the woman herself is seeing and feeling. In order to do that a lecture or a paper probably doesn't suffice, the midwives and doctors will close their ears to truths which are painful.

The most effective way that I have found so far of introducing midwives to what it is like for the woman going through their maternity services is to do a mini play. In the play I take on the role of a young girl of about 19 who lives in the most poverty-stricken area they can think of. My knowledge of childbirth is confined to an article I read in *Best* magazine, my boyfriend takes off when my pregnancy is confirmed, but he does come back further on during the pregnancy, I have had a row with my Mum because of the pregnancy and her disapproval of my boyfriend so at the beginning of the mini play I am very much alone.

As the play progresses I persuade about 35 midwives to arrange themselves in a long line on the stage and then I use them as characters in the play, so that the first person in the line is my GP to whom I report my pregnancy right at the beginning, the second person is the hospital receptionist to whom I take my letter, the third person is the midwife in the Clinic who books me, the fourth person is the doctor who examines me and so we go on. After having seen about 20 different midwives and doctors throughout my pregnancy I go into labour. During the labour the staff change at 8-hourly intervals and as I approach 8 cm dilatation the staff change again, in the throes of pain and transition I freak out, begging for a general anaesthetic, epidural, anything to help me with the pain – often this rather dramatic scene moves some of the audience to tears as they remember occasions when this happened to them or when they identify with the pain and despair of the young woman.

As we progress to the Postnatal Ward everyone realises that I have seen the whole 35 care-givers and we haven't included the domestics, the nursery nurses, the auxiliaries, etc. The whole mini play makes some of the audience very angry as they insist that it isn't like that for women where they work – I query this statement and ask them to do me a favour by just going back and looking at the notes of the first five women they come across in the Postnatal Ward and count the number of signatures.

The efficacy of this was demonstrated very strongly to me at the presentation I gave at the Westminster Hospital when the whole suggestion that women could see so many people was angrily rejected 'Because it's such a small Unit here'.

The Antenatal Clinic Sister told me that it was quite impossible for women to meet so many different people because it was only a small hospital and that they really did not have that number of doctors or midwives on the staff. I was prepared for this criticism and I had photocopied onto acetates ten antenatal records that I had found at random during visits to the wards the previous day. All I needed to show the midwives and the Antenatal Clinic Sister was the number of signatures, during the antenatal period alone, on each woman's notes. It was quite obvious that when women said that they saw a different person every time they were not mistaken, they really were seeing a different person every time and when they went into labour, even the people they had met before were not around, they met even more people – yet more strange midwives and doctors. I always have found this is a very salutary way of looking at one's service, just by looking at the different signatures in notes makes it absolutely apparent that women really do see an inordinate number of different people during their pregnancy, labour and puerperium.

Working as a Change Management Consultant

Because of the openness and the breadth of vision of the Director of Midwifery Services in Riverside Health Authority, Suzanne Truttero, a Change Management Consultant (myself) was appointed in order to initiate change. This meant that staff already working in the Unit could be helped, supported and guided through change rather than having to fit it in with their regular work.

At the time this was an unusual appointment. For most midwives trying to achieve change they will not be in such an advantageous position and will be having to achieve change as well as run the labour ward, deliver babies and work out next month's off duty.

If I describe the methods I used to achieve the changes within Riverside Health Authority, it must be acknowledged that this was done under ideal conditions – in a post expressly for bringing about such change, with supportive management, in a hospital about to close so that major change was in the background all the time. You may be fortunate in having such a post, but I suspect this is unlikely so we must also look at ways of achieving change when you are 'just' a student, or 'just' an ordinary midwife, undoubtedly more difficult but achievable none the less.

A step by step approach

Change needs to be achieved step by step. The post of Change Management Consultant enabled me to devote my time entirely to the two objectives I was detailed to achieve:

1. To increase continuity of care for women.
2. To increase the midwives' job satisfaction.

I had no other tasks to do, no other distractions, no other jobs. I worked 3 days a week or up to 12 days per month to achieve these two aims.

First of all I needed to get to know everybody, this entailed literally just walking around and getting to know everybody's name and everybody's face and helping them to get to know me and to get to know my face. In part this was forced upon us because it took a month before an office was found for me and Janet Andrews, who was (and is) the person who works as my secretary, assistant, organiser and friend and supporter. So Janet's and my first role was that of peripatetics in that we roamed around the Maternity Unit getting to know people.

In order to help people to get to know me and also to open their minds to self publicity I sent round a card, with a photograph of myself on the front and details of myself and my family and the reason I was at the Westminster Hospital, to all members of the Midwifery Staff. I wanted them to see how this increased their knowledge of me so that they could become familiar with this way of learning about people. In the future I was hoping to increase the women's knowledge of the midwives and by doing this it helped the midwives to have some experience of seeing a photograph of somebody and learning their details.

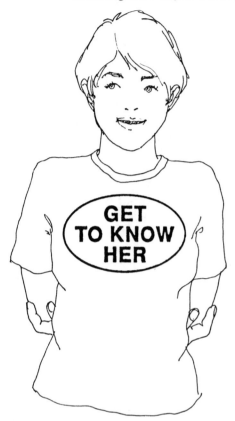

Once Janet and I had an office where we could actually hang
our coats and fix up our computer and photocopier I began to
do a survey of the women being looked after in the hospital. I
asked them what it was like having a baby in the Westminster
Hospital. Despite general satisfaction with the care they were
receiving they told me that there were long waits at the
Antenatal Clinic and that they met different people every time
they came. What they wanted above all was the same person to
look after them throughout their pregnancy and who would
also be with them during their labour.

While I was surveying the women I was also surveying the
midwives, the hospital doctors, the health visitors and the GPs.
The midwives were mainly happy working in the Westminster
Hospital but they found it difficult that their off duty was only
done about a fortnight in advance, and they would have

preferred to know their off duty further in advance. They also would have liked to provide continuity of care for the women they were looking after. For the midwives as well it was difficult working in such a fragmented way.

Surveying the hospital doctors was interesting in that their concerns were the smooth running of the whole Unit, they were angry that pathology investigations took a long time to come back, or that the Antenatal Clinic did not run smoothly, I realised that their view was much more global than was the midwives' or the women's. The GPs in the area that I spoke to felt that the communications with the Hospital were poor and they wanted to know more about what was happening to their patients during their pregnancies.

Having roamed around for about 2 months making notes, interviewing and talking with people, I then did some presentations – two during the daytime and one at night. The presentation aimed to show the midwives and doctors the results of my surveys – what it was like for women who came to the Hospital. As described before, I lined up 35 members of the audience in a row and I showed them graphically what it was like for a woman who came to the Antenatal Clinic for the first time and met a midwife and a doctor, and then when she came a second time she met another midwife and another doctor. The third time she met yet another midwife and yet another doctor and so on and so on. I showed them that many women were meeting 35 to 40 different midwives and doctors during their time at the Westminster Hospital.

Midwives began to see what really happened to women in their Unit – they began to see that a change in the way the care was given was necessary.

Setting up an Action Group

The next step was to set up an Action Group to meet every week. The purpose of this Action Group was to enable those attending to get to know each other and for them to then explore how the problems that we had could be overcome. In order to change a service it seemed more sensible to get the people working inside the system to suggest changes then, hopefully, they would feel that the ideas were their own and would be willing to implement them.

Every member of the Midwifery and Medical Staff was invited to the weekly Action Groups and every member of the Midwifery and Medical Staff received Minutes of the Action Group. Between Action Group meetings I went round and talked to the Staff who did not attend the Action Group meeting to find out how they felt and to have their input.

The Action Group meetings were held very early in the mornings before the day staff began or at the end of the afternoon shift or during the afternoon overlap. The times of the meetings were varied so that people could come if they were on different shifts. The meetings were exciting, some people came to every single meeting whether they were off duty or not and other people came just once or twice. I tried to make the meetings exciting and interesting, and I tried very hard to make the midwives feel very welcome. We always offered tea and coffee and delicious biscuits.

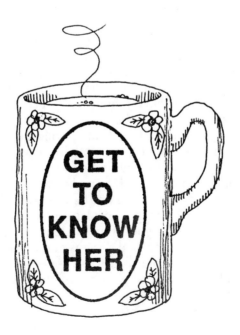

Invitations to these Action Group meetings included Obstetricians, Midwives, NCT members, Health Visitors, GPs – in fact anyone who was interested.

Over a period of 9 months, 16 meetings of the Action Group were held. Discussions and suggestions ranged over the central problems which were perceived to be:

1. Lack of continuity of care of women.
2. Poor communications with GPs.
3. Poor communications with Health Visitors.
4. Midwives wanting to know their off duties more than a fortnight in advance.

Many different ways of working in order to overcome these difficulties were discussed. Where care should be based was addressed – it seemed sensible that as women lived in the community and spent most of their pregnancy, some of their labour and all of the time with their baby there in the community, that care should be based in the community.

One of the most important parts of the Action Group was for people to get to know each other. There was a distinct reluctance to get to know each other better because everybody assured me that they already knew each other. However, it was interesting that when I insisted that everyone in the room should say what their name was and secondly tell us something good and something bad that had happened to them since we last met, it was extraordinary how many people said "Oh I never knew that about you" when they learnt that a colleague's husband was chronically ill or that a colleague was having problems with her housing or some other aspect of her life.

It would seem to me that we must work better and more happily if we know that our colleagues know us and care about what is going on in our lives. No one had to say more than they were prepared to, some people decided to be quite flippant in what they revealed: "The good thing is that I managed to get out of bed this morning, the bad thing is that it isn't my day off until Friday". Other people were very honest with their concerns in life and the midwives really got to know each other and to function as a team.

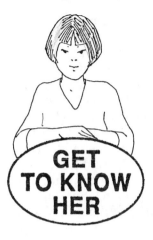

Human beings are so attractive to each other that when they get to know each other well, they begin to love each other and care about each other and give greater consideration to each other. If we just do not know our colleagues it is exceedingly difficult for us to get to know them well or to care about them. If we do not feel cared about ourselves it is very difficult for us to care about other people and so give good care to the women we are looking after.

The Action Groups explored how everybody would ideally like to work. Our aims were: to increase continuity of carer for women; to increase the job satisfaction of the midwives; to improve communications with the GPs, and to provide a dynamic and excellent service for all people in the Health Authority. We explored midwives having their own caseload, and there were some enthusiastic members of the group who would have liked to have their own caseload and to look after antenatally, deliver and look after postnatally only those women on their caseload. They talked about it and investigated how it would be and how many women they could take on, but in the end they decided that it was not the way they wanted to work, they wanted to be sure of their days off every week. They did not want their holidays to be interrupted. They wanted to know that when they were off duty they really were off duty and not likely to be called to somebody in labour.

Next we began to explore not just one person having a caseload but two or three midwives sharing a caseload. This computation was explored and then rejected because the off duty didn't seem very attractive. The Group ended up by deciding that six midwives in a Team meant that all midwives got every alternate weekend off and they only had to be on call for seven periods of 24 hours in 5 weeks, and that sounded very good. We worked out dozens of off duties and we looked at the Health Authority's geography and divided it up into patches which were co-terminous with the Health Visitors and decided that this was the way that the midwives would like to work.

During my surveying period I had met several of the Health Visitors in the district. For them the main problem that they highlighted was the poor relationship they had with the Community Midwives, they felt that they were frequently not given information that was necessary for effectively carrying out their work.

The obvious way to overcome this problem, and to help Midwives and Health Visitors to work better together, was to have them working from the same place and perhaps – even better – to have them working from the same office where they could see each other frequently. Communications couldn't help but improve if they were all making tea from the same kettle and sharing the same desks.

We continued to explore how the teams of six could work. We wrote a proposal detailing the suggested way of working that we had decided upon. I spent a considerable amount of time talking to all those people who never came to meetings. One group I found extremely difficult were the night staff, many of whom had been working at night for many years. Many of them were welcoming and pleasant but there was a core of midwives working at night who were extremely unwelcoming to me when I turned up (having telephoned first) during the night, I found myself more and more reluctant to go in at night. First of all having to haul oneself out of bed very early in the morning was never pleasant, and then to be greeted by scowls and people being 'too busy' to speak to you (even when there was no labouring woman in sight), was extremely difficult. I was to find later that the antagonism of the night staff was extremely destructive and, in retrospect, I think I should have worked harder to encourage them to give their suggestions and ideas and perhaps have tried to be less sensitive to their lack of welcome.

Looking back it is obvious that those people who never attend a meeting, despite receiving minutes and invitations to all the meetings, are making as strong a statement when they don't come to meetings as those who enthusiastically turn up at every meeting. In retrospect I could have been more aware of that and I should have pursued midwives more to find out their opinions and feelings about the proposals. In fairness I did try and pursue people as much as possible, but it was always difficult and was invariably the task I put off until last on the days when I was working. Some people would literally 'disappear' when I arrived on their ward; having been obviously visible only seconds before my arrival in, for instance, the Antenatal Clinic, they were nowhere to be seen once I arrived. At first I accepted this but eventually I realised that it always happened with specific people and that they had got 'disappearing' down to an art form!

All the time the Action Groups were meeting I also pursued the Consultant Obstetricians, making sure that they had read the minutes coming out from the Action Group and finding out their reactions to them, and to gather their suggestions.

The most difficult group to liaise with was the GPs. At first I wrote to each GP telling him why I had been appointed and asking for a meeting with him/her to discuss the proposals and to get his/her input and suggestions. Trying to get through to them on the telephone to follow up my letter was very hard – either the surgery was closed (every surgery appeared to have different opening hours to every other) and an answering machine told me the emergency number. When I was eventually able to get through the receptionist invariably found it difficult to know why someone who wasn't a patient was ringing the doctor, after a severe quizzing I was finally able to make an appointment with the GP. When I arrived the GP was frequently delayed, had slipped out for a quick bit of shopping or had forgotten our appointment or had been called away.

Despite the frustration incurred by most of my GP visits some of them were wonderful, they had arranged lunches with all the Partners and the Health Visitor there. Some were already doing wonderful and imaginative schemes for the women in their area, but most were just plodding along and providing a minimum service of shared antenatal care for the women. They complained about the lack of communication from the Hospital and they approved of the notion that more care should be carried out in the community but they did not perceive that there could be any change in how the care they provided was given and they all told me that their patients enjoyed their antenatal care from them. When asked if they would like to become more involved in intrapartum care, or even to just 'pop in' and give the woman a few words of comfort during labour in the Hospital which was very nearby, they invariably felt that they would not have time.

Twenty-four GP surgeries were visited, the plans and ideas were discussed with them – most were fairly enthusiastic, most felt that they were giving women an excellent service already but felt unable (except for one) to offer any intrapartum care or even a visit in labour. One particular group stated quite categorically that all their women wanted to go to St Thomas's Hospital and this is where they sent all their patients. Many of the GPs wanted an attached midwife to do their antenatal care for or with them, they felt that she could then do all the deliveries if she was willing.

A difference in perceptions about involvement in birth

There was a lack of understanding about the amount of flexibility and commitment it would take for one midwife to be involved in all the deliveries from one practice, but this was probably understandable.

For a woman and her husband labour is a period which lasts 24–36 hours continuously.

For a doctor the same labour will represent perhaps a couple of visits during that time and then a concerted period of about 45 minutes at the birth of the baby, because the continuous care will be given by a midwife.

For a midwife the same labour represents the same period of time that it does for the parents, except that at the beginning of it she will offer one or two visits and then when it becomes established she will stay with the couple continuously. This period of time extends much longer than the actual birth of the baby or even the delivery of the placenta because for the midwife it includes writing the notes, putting them on the computer, informing the GP/Paediatrician/Supervisor of Midwives, bathing the mother, helping with the feeding of the baby, settling the mother and baby down afterwards and cleaning and clearing up the room. Most of which are tasks which escape the doctor.

Negotiations

Throughout this period I discovered who were members of the Local Medical Group, who was in the Division of Obstetrics, who was the Chair of the Division. A lot of time was spent lobbying GPs and Obstetricians, so that when these meetings happened several key people at the meeting would be supportive of the suggestions. I had learnt from bitter experience that this does not just happen within the NHS; it is essential that one goes and talks to all the people who are likely to be at a meeting so that they feel a specific interest in the project because you have approached them about it. It cannot, even if it is the most sensible idea in the world, be left to chance because in the NHS, perhaps because it is a large and amorphous body, people need to be shown personally what the suggestion is before they can actually see clearly the proposal that you are making.

All the lobbying and the meeting of different people took an inordinate amount of time. It was essential that I had an assistant as competent as Janet Andrews who could get the minutes out, buy the biscuits for the meetings, put notices up in the wards about different meetings, and generally keep the whole show going. It seems to me that this would have been an impossible task if I had been a senior midwife with no secretarial help supposed to be doing all my other work as well.

As you will see from the preceding paragraphs most of my job was liaison and public relations. The aim was that everybody would feel part of the changes and developments that were happening within Riverside Health Authority. It was rumoured that the Westminster Hospital Maternity Unit would be closing so the midwives felt insecure and sad about this; we settled down to find better ways of giving care and making something very sad into a positive move which would provide better care for the women of Riverside Health Authority.

The first draft proposal

After four meetings the Action Group formulated a draft proposal for working with four Teams in the Community. This was sent to every midwife (posted to her home address) working in the Health Authority for her comments and suggestions – each midwife was interviewed to ascertain her preference for working in the Hospital or the Community. Staff satisfaction questionnaires were given out to all midwives; these were to be compared with staff satisfaction questionnaires to be given out as the schemes developed.

The draft proposal suggested four Teams of midwives working in the East side of Riverside Health Authority to work in a geographical location, alongside Health Visitors. They would be based in the same Health Authority buildings as the Health Visitors.

The first draft proposal also went to every member of the Obstetric Staff, very few comments came back but those that did were quite comprehensive so the third draft of the proposal looked very different from the first draft. The proposal was taken to the Local Medical Group and was approved, having been discussed with key members before it actually came to the Group. The proposal went to the Division of Obstetrics and was also passed at that meeting.

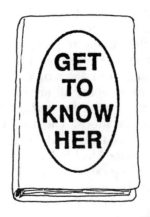

The proposal then went to the Health Authority where it was introduced by the Chair of the Maternity Services Liaison Committee, who was a lay woman who had a huge interest in the Maternity Services and was exceedingly dynamic and astute in the local political sphere. Once it had got through all the committees and was to be put into place the news came through that the Westminster Hospital Maternity Unit was definitely going to close and so the Midwifery Management Team decided that the Teams of six midwives based in the community would start on 1 February 1989. This left little time to prepare for the massive change, but it felt exceedingly positive that we had a starting date.

The next action was to interview every midwife and find out where she felt her skills were lacking and where she specifically felt she needed to spend some time. Was it in the Antenatal Clinic to learn the procedure and tests that were carried out at the Booking Visit? Was it in the Labour Ward to brush up on delivery techniques? Was it in the Postnatal Ward to find out how to put a woman on the computer who was being discharged? Every midwife had different needs for updating.

Applications were invited for members of the four teams of six midwives who would be working in the community. Since whispers of what we were doing had got out there had been many midwives who applied for jobs on the Teams from both inside and outside the Hospital. Finally 24 midwives were appointed who were to become the first four Teams of six. My work was then to train and prepare the Teams and the people they were to work with.

In order to publicise their work and to help women to get to know them each midwife gave me a photograph and a short description of herself, her interests and hobbies, and these were put in a description of each member making up a Team.

Training sessions were held with the Teams and the Health Visitors they were to work with, usually on the site where they were to be based. The sessions with the Health Visitors were 'getting to know each other' sessions and visualising how the Team would work in the Health Authority hospital building, how it would liaise with the Health Visitors, how they would work together, what time they would come in in the morning, what time they would leave, what time they would go off duty, the mechanisms they would employ to ensure that communications with the Health Visitors ran smoothly and generally visualising how they were going to work and what the Health Visitors' needs were as well as theirs.

Often the Teams were put into very small spaces because all the Health Authority buildings were lacking in space, and once it was realised that the Teams would actually take up physical space they were less popular than they had been when they had just been a twinkle in somebody's eye!

As many workshops as possible were held, each one was an exercise in getting to know each other – learning about the important things in each others' lives, the interests, the family, the pets, the hopes and aspirations of each Team member. The principle was that human beings are naturally attracted to each other, the more they know about each other, the better they know each other, the more they can empathise with each other and support each other when working together.

Getting to know you games

Opening gambits were used such as:

- Something good and something bad that has happened to me since we last met.
- Something different about me that is different from everybody else in the room.
- What I hope to be doing in 5 years' time.
- What I would be doing if it was my day off today.
- The most important thing in my life.
- What I do when I am having fun.
- What I would be doing if I wasn't here.
- What I would do if I won the pools.

Visualising how the teams would work

The workshops with the Teams of midwives themselves consisted of a great many 'getting to know each other' exercises.

A difficult exercise was visualising how the midwives would be working. It was important for them to realise the amount of disorientation, shock and distress they would experience when working in a totally different environment. The Community Midwives would not find it so disorientating working in the community, but they too would be working in a totally different way from the way they had been working before and they would also experience distress and disorientation. When a Hospital Midwife comes on duty at 7.30 a.m., she knows that she is going to go off duty at about 4.30 p.m., she knows that it is the medicine round at 10 a.m. and 2 p.m., she knows that she will first of all have the report and then she will go round and see the women and pick up specific things to do. She knows that the nappies are kept in this cupboard and the MSU packs are kept in that cupboard, and that lunch will arrive at 12.30. There are certain basics which always happen and always have happened and that she is familiar with, when she goes off duty she is aware of what she has done and how the day has progressed.

The midwives working in the Teams were to work in a totally different way. First, every day would be different and there would be no boundaries. The midwives themselves would have to get together the MSU packs, the sphygmomanometers, the pinards stethoscopes; each individual midwife had to make it her responsibility that she had the right equipment. The Senior Midwives would order what was needed but they needed to know what to order. The midwives were given dockets so that they could go and buy themselves bags at a local department store. Some paid extra and had very exciting bags, others had more mundane bags, very few midwives had the same bag as anybody else.

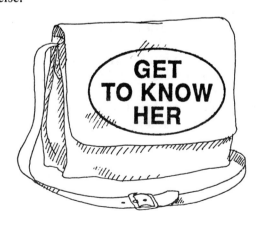

The midwives needed to set up their office, to discuss and decide where they were going to keep their paper, their notes, their inco pads. Because the Westminster Hospital Maternity Unit was closing down it was possible to obtain office equipment that was no longer to be used. Chairs and desks were available, and all these were transported to the Local Authority buildings where the midwives were going to work. The midwives began to realise that they were going to be in charge of their off duty and when the work had finished for the day they would go home, there would be no one to say to them 'go home', they themselves would have to decide this. It sounded easy, but when it came to it this was one of the most difficult things for a midwife to do, especially if for a couple of days she had very little to do, midwives felt guilty about going home and were frightened that the hospital would take back hours that they felt that they 'owed', so that often the midwives would turn up in the Labour Ward to help because they found it difficult to allow themselves not to work even though there was actually no work to be done.

The off duties were devised so that when a midwife was on call she was only on call, no other work input was expected of her. Later on this was to change slightly in that a midwife who was on call and had been on call for several days and had not been called would offer to help her colleagues with antenatal and postnatal visits or with bookings, so that she did do the requisite number of hours each month.

The Midwife Managers got together the equipment each Team needed, car leasing was sorted out, midwives decided on whether they were going to use bicycles, taxis or cars. Midwife Managers decided on the scale of the allowances and how much it would cost.

Publicity was organised. The photographs of the midwives with details of their hobbies and interests were gathered together and an information sheet was made up for each Team which gave the address of their Clinic, the contact number for their bleep and the details and pictures of all the members of the Teams.

The start of the Community Teams

The Community Teams started work on Monday 6 February 1989. On the Sunday prior to that, each midwife received her kit and a handbook written by the Change Management Consultant to help them with their new roles. The Westminster Hospital Maternity Unit closed with only a few women in the Postnatal Ward – the wards were staffed until all the women had gone home, so by the end of the week the whole Unit had closed. There were 24 midwives in the Teams and there were two Community Midwives who had refused to join the Teams, their brief was to look after women who had gone to hospitals outside the district who needed postnatal care and also to look after those women who had had private obstetric care and needed postnatal visiting.

One of the most important instructions to all the Teams was that they should have a weekly meeting. At this they all got together in order to get to know each other better and discuss how they were working and what improvements/changes they wanted to make. At these meetings the Senior Midwife for the Community or sometimes I went. It was important that the Teams should have support and encouragement because the transition from hospital to working in the Community as a Team Midwife was exceedingly difficult, and indeed the midwives did feel very disorientated and confused during this time. First, there were articles of equipment that the midwives had forgotten to provide themselves with, so those needed acquiring. Then the right forms were not available so those needed chasing up. A mechanism had to be put in place by which the Team Midwives could be informed about women in their area. We were lucky to have a member of the Medical Records Department, Carole Croxall, who took on all the medical records for Team Midwifery and who organised referrals to the Team Midwives.

Whenever a GP wrote to refer a woman to the hospital (now the West London Hospital), Carole Croxall made out a set of notes for that woman and sent the notes to the Team Midwives in their respective Health Authority buildings.

The Team Midwives would decide when they would go to the woman's home to do a booking and the woman received a letter with a 'Team Sheet' which consisted of six photographs depicting each member of the Midwifery Team and a few personal details about her. It also had the telephone number that the woman needed to ring in order to bleep the midwife who was on call for that day. Women were instructed that they could bleep the number any time of the day or night and they would get through to one of the six midwives. The midwives wrote to the women to say that they would be coming to do a Booking Visit on a certain day and at a certain time and if this day and time were not convenient the woman was to ring their telephone number and make a date with the midwives which was more convenient to her. The midwife then went to the woman's home and did her Booking Visit and took her Booking bloods and arranged with her the pattern of her future antenatal care.

The fly in the ointment was (and is) the processing of blood results. In London there are private laboratories and if you use them you are supplied with Freepost labels and padded envelopes and these specimens are just placed inside a postbox and the results come back a few days later. The Health Authority system was not as efficient as this and bloods needed to be transported to a main collecting point, such as a clinic or hospital when they were picked up, sometimes lost, and the results took quite a while to be returned.

The Booking notes were discussed with one of the obstetricians or a registrar, in order to ensure that the midwives had made the right decisions with that specific woman and had not missed any complications. This system was eventually to go by default, mainly because the consultant obstetrician was not available or because the midwives were too busy, and also because the obstetricians realised that the midwives were not trying to stop high-risk women from seeing them, but were dealing appropriately and sensibly with all women. So some women were never to see anybody but a midwife, some women whose GPs specifically requested were to see only a midwife but also their GP on one, two or three occasions. Some women were to see an obstetrician once, some women were never to see an obstetrician, and other women who were high risk were to see an obstetrician on alternate visits and the midwives on the intervening visits. Each woman had a programme that she had discussed with a midwife and which was appropriate to her level of need. These schedules were to be changed if circumstances changed. It seemed to work well.

The midwives started by doing postnatal care for the women in their area, but these were women they had never met before and so as well as feeling disorientated because their working day had changed so radically they were also not having any of the satisfaction that continuity of carer brings. I kept re-iterating this to them and kept urging them to be patient because eventually they would see the benefits of working in this way, but I told them time after time that it would be at least 3 or 4 months before they experienced the pleasure of continuity of carer.

The difficulty of being a pioneer cannot be overstated. There are no walls, no edges to the range of experience, people experiencing such radical change feel exhausted, depressed and confused. Even in a job that is boring and lacking in satisfaction you know when you clock on, when you clock off and what you will be doing during the hours you are there. There is structure.

The Community Teams had no structure at the beginning – they had to define it themselves, check it out with each other and then make it Team practice. When each thing has to be gone through in this way it is utterly exhausting.

The Midwifery Consultant sent several encouraging letters, the Teams Manager Yvonne Stone spent time with each Team and each Team member – encouraging and supporting. It could never be enough, even with support and care the Team members found it very hard, but they persevered, shape began to emerge, order began to come out of chaos, they began to grow into cohesive Teams – not always successfully. One Team has been known to pick on its newer or less confident members and to make life very hard for them; in fact one Team has received counselling on its interaction.

Light at the end of the tunnel

Eventually the women began to bleep the midwives when they were in labour and the midwives at last began to deliver women they knew. They then carried out postnatal care on women they had delivered. The change was electric. Midwives began to see how the scheme would work and they began to see what it was like to get to know a woman and to look after her during this important time in her life.

The Teams bringing women into the Hospital began to feel the full wrath of the Hospital Midwives. The Teams were scapegoated for all the ills of the Hospital merger. The Westminster Hospital Maternity Unit had closed and the midwives who had not gone on the Community Teams transferred to the West London Hospital – every time a Community Team Midwife brought a woman into the labour ward there were grumbles. Either she hadn't left the room clean enough, or the Hospital staff had not relieved her for coffee or meal breaks, or she hadn't consulted the doctors in the right way, or she hadn't said good morning cheerfully enough.

The problem was that the midwives who were being incorporated into the West London hated the changes. The West London midwives hated having to incorporate all these strange midwives. In retrospect the overriding need was for there to be 'getting to know you' exercises carried out at that stage for all the midwives working within the hospital, but the setting up of the Community Teams took a great deal of thought and energy and none was left over for the Hospital set up.

During July 1989 a questionnaire to assess the satisfaction levels of midwives working in the Community Teams was sent out. The overall result was that although starting the Teams had been very hard, the result of working within them had been very stimulating and satisfying for the midwives involved – their confidence had increased dramatically, they enjoyed being able to practise their role to the full, they loved being able to get to know the women throughout their pregnancy and then to go on to look after them in labour and deliver them, and finally to watch and support the emergence of a new family.

There have been problems for the Teams – some GPs have been particularly uncooperative, sending their patients to St Thomas's Hospital in order to circumvent the Team system. Each midwife in each Team has a certain number of GPs allocated to her and her remit is to liaise with those GPs and communicate with them so that problems are averted and so that they know what is going on with their patients – this works to a greater or lesser extent – often lesser unfortunately, GPs are concerned that they may lose the not inconsiderable financial remuneration they get from maternity care. They also don't always trust midwives' clinical judgement, despite the fact that midwives have received at least 18 months' specialist training in their field and doctors have usually at the very most received 6 months' specialist training.

The future

Now after 3½ years this way of working seems very usual and permanent for most of the midwives in the Teams. There are still problems and frustrations with the way Teams work – the problems with blood results have never been resolved, there is still some griping and bitching from Hospital Midwives, but on the whole the Hospital Team Midwives get on very well with their attached Community Team and often offer them support and help.

A question still remaining is whether the Community Teams would work better with a Team Leader – most of the Teams seem to work very happily together but sometimes there appears to be a place for someone to be in charge – the philosophy is that this happens naturally which it probably does most of the time.

Another question is whether the Teams need clerical support – in an ideal world probably the answer is yes, in an NHS which is being run down this is probably impossible, but this is the type of Health Care Assistant most of the Teams would appreciate.

The Community Team Midwives mostly enjoy working in the way that they do – the most common refrain from them is that if they ever want to move out of London where on earth can they move to? They are unanimous that they could never bear to work in any other way after having worked in a Community Team.

How can I achieve change?

It's all very well talking about how to achieve change when you have had the privilege of being appointed specifically to achieve change within a Unit, but how does somebody who is working as a Student Midwife or as a Staff Midwife or as a Midwifery Sister in a Unit achieve change?

Sometimes the answer is that she just can't and it is impossible, but in several Units, Team schemes and continuity of carer schemes have come about because of the persistence and enthusiasm of one Staff Midwife or one Midwifery Sister who has encouraged, cajoled, made a nuisance of themselves and generally pushed the rest of the Unit towards initiating the sort of changes they were looking for. How do these people go about it, how can an isolated person in a humble position change the way women have babies in that area?

First, it is probably helpful if she writes down what her objectives are, what she actually wants to achieve. How she wants to see her Unit working in 5 years time. Then she needs to approach those people who will be sympathetic and 'on her side'. If these people have fairly powerful positions that is all to the better, for instance the Professor of Obstetrics or one of the Obstetricians. If you are in a fairly lowly position you may be intimidated at the very thought of approaching such august beings but you will be surprised that if you say you want to talk about something with them, and if you ask if you can make an appointment to talk with them for just 20 minutes about new ways of developing the care given in your Unit, they will usually be very sympathetic and welcoming.

If you can then write down what you envisage in no more than two or three pages then it is all to the better. Once you have seen two or three people you should start to produce a document of your thoughts – this will change and develop as people make suggestions and point out flaws. You will know if you observe closely, who holds the most power in your organisation – often it will not necessarily be the people one expects. It is often a good idea to approach different specialties. For instance having spoken to two of the Consultant Obstetricians and got their blessing it is now worth approaching the Clinical Director and then the Chief Midwife.

I wish I could say always approach the Chief Midwife first and that she will listen openly and enthusiastically to your ideas and will get them initiated. If you have that sort of Chief Midwife it is obvious that she is where you should go first. But if you do not have that sort of Chief Midwife and you feel she will either laugh at your ideas or ignore them then it is better to go to the Obstetricians first. It is also usually not very constructive to talk and chat with any group of midwives who are always complaining about management. If you want to do something positive you need to go about it in a very positive manner. Each time you approach a new person you can tell them about the other people you have approached. For instance you can say:

> I talked to Mr Johnston about this scheme and he was very enthusiastic and then I talked to Mrs Reagan and she also thought this was a very good idea. Next I went to the Professor and he thought it was a very good idea as long as we did a research project allied to it. Now I have come to you and am wondering what you feel about it and whether there is any possibility of us setting up an Action Group or Working Party to look into the feasibility of setting this up in our Unit.

If the answer is a blunt refusal you obviously haven't chosen the right people to go to, or maybe your Unit is a lost cause and you should consider moving house! Do not be discouraged, change always takes longer than you think. You will sometimes need to go back to the drawing board and think of another way of presenting your ideas. So this time you produce a research project which happens to include continuity of carer, and you find a new way of dressing up your original proposal. We never realise how long massive changes take, they never happen fast enough and for those of us who constantly think ahead and can't believe that everything happens so slowly it can be extremely frustrating.

Eventually with perseverance you will triumph. People move, people retire and eventually you will find that the plan which you tried to initiate 5 years ago or 3 years ago is now taking place. Often it is not seen as your idea nor does it always bear a very strong resemblance to your original plans. But as long as the basics are there and as long as women are being delivered by midwives they are getting to know, then you have triumphed and you have set up a way of birth for women that will give them great satisfaction and pleasure.

JUST KEEP TRYING

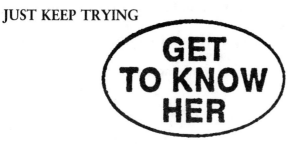

3

The research basis

Enthusiasts of continuity of carer list many benefits from being able to get to know a woman throughout her pregnancy, labour and postnatal period. The benefits which are cited are:

1. That women like it.
2. That midwives like it.
3. That there are fewer antenatal admissions thereby providing cost savings.
4. There are fewer forceps deliveries and caesarean sections and thereby cost savings.
5. There is less intervention such as acceleration of labour and induction of labour, thereby providing cost savings.
6. There are fewer Category X patients (women who go into the Labour Ward who are not in established labour, who are either sent home or, more frequently, sent to an Antenatal Ward or are induced because labour is not established).
7. That midwives learn better from seeing a woman all the way through her pregnancy, labour and the puerperium and by seeing the effects of her practice the midwife learns more.
8. That midwifery staff is utilised better and that midwives are where women are rather than staffing an area.
9. That midwives have increased job satisfaction.
10. That there are improved relationships between the midwives working in a Team.
11. There are improved relationships between the midwives and the mother.
12. That babies are bigger when their mothers have received care from known midwives.
13. That continuity of care from known midwives costs less.

Is there any research to either confirm or refute these assumptions?

As long ago as 1969 a randomised controlled trial of 1773 women was described in the bulletin of the American College of Nurse-Midwives. Seven hundred and sixty-eight women were randomised into care by nurse-midwives, and 1005 women were randomised to be cared for by physicians. Nurse-midwives gave more of the women they cared for analgesic drugs, but in smaller doses, and the women looked after by nurse-midwives had bigger babies, shorter total length of labours and shorter second stage of labours. Ninety-three percent of the women looked after by nurse-midwives had normal deliveries compared with 41% of women who were looked after by physicians. Fifty-eight percent of the physicians' patients had operative deliveries compared with 2% of the nurse-midwives' patients. The women who were attended by physicians were looked after in the way normally practised in the United States of America – they are looked after by doctors rather than midwives, who are in exceedingly short supply in the United States of America (in many states midwifery is illegal).

Another randomised controlled trial was described by Slome *et al.* in the *American Journal of Obstetrics and Gynecology* in 1976, where 438 women were randomised into two groups, one of 298 women who were cared for by nurse-midwives and 140 women who were cared for by physicians during 1973 and 1974. The women looked after by nurse-midwives kept 94% of their antenatal appointments, whereas women looked after by physicians only kept 80% of their antenatal appointments. The women looked after by certified nurse-midwives had an 82.6% normal delivery rate compared to women looked after by physicians who had a 2.1% normal delivery rate. Of the women looked after by certified nurse-midwives, 9.1% had a forceps delivery, compared with 29.5% of the women looked after by physicians.

In a randomised controlled trial the women are selected because of matching characteristics and then they are randomised into two groups, so the women in these trials should all have been very similar in such characteristics as level of risk and previous pregnancy history etc. Therefore with both these trials the difference in the outcome for the women is specifically because of the treatment they received from the different personnel rather than in any characteristic of the women.

Karen Kowalski, Gottschalk, Greer and others (1977) looked at a scheme instituted at the University of Colorado Medical Center to:

1. Alleviate lack of continuity of care of obstetric patients.
2. Counter inadequate prenatal instruction.
3. Alleviate the unpredictability of patient sensors in the labour and delivery area.

Four Teams of two nurses each were given a caseload and gave antenatal care to women. When women went into labour one of their nurses was called and looked after them in labour and then saw the women every day while they were in the Postnatal Ward (but this was for only a very short time because women stayed in for only a day or two). One hundred women who had been looked after by the nurse partnerships were compared with 500 women in a control group. There was no significant difference in infant or maternal mortality or morbidity and there was no difference in the length of labour. There were, however, differences found, in that women looked after by nurse partnerships had fewer visits to the hospital in false labour or to the Hospital Accident and Emergency Unit for complications and problems. The women who had been looked after by one of the nurse partnerships expressed greater satisfaction and there was a significant decrease in the complaints regarding the obstetric service from women who had been looked after by the nurse partnerships.

In 1981, Doris Haire wrote an article in the *Journal of Nurse-Midwifery* about the North Central Bronx Hospital (Haire, 1981), in which she quoted the figures for 1979, when there were 2608 deliveries in this hospital. The hospital is situated in one of the most sociologically depressed areas of New York where mothers are predominantly black, hispanic or poor white women. Thirty per cent of the women are characterised as high risk due to poverty and drug useage. Because the Hospital was in such a poverty-stricken area it was exceedingly unpopular with doctors and most of the care in the hospital was given by midwives. Eighty-three percent of the women were delivered by midwives and in 1979 the hospital had an 88% normal delivery rate. Ninety-three percent of babies weighing more than 1000 g had Apgar scores of more than 7, analgesia was used in less than 30% of labours, the caesarean section rate was 9% and the instrumental delivery rate was 2.3%. This, in a country which is (and was then) renowned for its very high caesarean section rates and low normal delivery rates, made fascinating reading.

Another article in the *Journal of Nurse-Midwifery* by Stein in 1986 reported a study held between 1974 and 1984, when 89 women whose babies presented by the breech at term were managed by using a Team approach between the nurse-midwives and the physicians. Eighty-nine women presented at 37 weeks' gestation or greater with a singleton fetus in the breech presentation were managed by nurse-midwives. It was described by the doctors that they had "extended the professional courtesy of delivering the breech infant" to their colleagues, the nurse-midwives.

- 62 (69.6%) of the women were having their first babies.
- 27 (30.3%) of the women were having their second or subsequent babies.
- 32 (36%) of the women had vaginal births and 57 (64%) of the women had caesarean births.

Although a fairly small study, it is interesting in that physicians in such a litigation-conscious country as the United States felt able to trust and rely on midwives in this way.

Marianne Biro and Judith Lumley wrote up the outcomes from the Monash Birth Centre in the *Medical Journal of Australia* in 1991. The Monash Birth Centre has strict selection criteria and in the period described 3085 women were booked for delivery in the Unit, of those 89 women went into labour or miscarried before 20 weeks and 138 withdrew at their own request to seek an alternative form of care. The 2858 remaining women gave birth to 2874 babies. The study looks at the perinatal mortality rate and birth weight of the babies and concluded that team midwifery as practised at the Monash Birth Centre was as safe as the standard maternity care provided within the State.

The Institute of Nursing at the Radcliffe Infirmary in Oxford evaluated the implementation of the Kidlington Team Midwifery Scheme and reported an increase in job satisfaction for midwives working in a Team providing continuity of carer and an increase in satisfaction of women (Kidlington Midwifery Scheme, 1990). Women looked after by midwives who they had been able to get to know used less analgesia during labour and had more positive comments than the women in the Control group. There were no differences in obstetric outcome for either mother or babies.

Know Your Midwife scheme

The Know Your Midwife research has already been quoted elsewhere, this was a randomised controlled trial of 1001 low-risk pregnant women, half of whom were offered Know Your Midwife care by a Team of four midwives. For those women the benefits were that they felt more in control of their labour (shown at 6 weeks postnatally), they felt all the choices had been explained to them in labour (shown at 6 weeks postnatally), they felt very well prepared for looking after a baby and they found it easier being a mother (shown at 6 weeks postnatally). Those being looked after by a Know Your Midwife Team found it easier to discuss anxieties in the clinic and found the midwives very helpful with their anxieties. Although the difference in antenatal admissions was not statistically significant there was a difference between the two groups in that the control groups spent 155 more days in hospital antenatally than did the experimental group. If the cost of a day in a London teaching hospital is in the region of £200, this represented a cost saving over 2 years of £31 000.

Other cost-saving aspects of care were a statistically significant difference in that 71.8% of the Know Your Midwife women went into spontaneous labour compared with only 62% of the control group, and fewer women in the Know Your Midwife group had accelerated and induced labours. More women in the Know Your Midwife Group had no analgesia or only Entonox. There were cost savings implicated by the fact that only 18.3% of the women having Know Your Midwife care had epidurals compared with 30.2% of women in the control group, and there were more normal deliveries in primigravid women than there were in the control group although this was not statistically significant. The number of episiotomies in primigravid women was highly statistically significant – only 46.5% of the women in the Know Your

Midwife group had an episiotomy compared to 62.3% in the control group. Were the babies bigger when their mothers had been looked after by known midwives? The mean birthweight of babies born to Know Your Midwife mothers was 3.284 kg whilst the mean birthweight of babies born to women in the Control Group was 3.218 kg, but this was not statistically significant.

Although no survey was done of staff satisfaction of the Know Your Midwife Team, the Director of Midwifery Services sent questionnaires to 208 members of staff which included Consultants, Junior Medical Staff, Midwifery Tutors, Midwifery Managers and Midwifery Sisters and Staff Midwives, to ask how they felt the pilot scheme was working and whether they would be willing to participate in a similar scheme. The response rate was 75.6% and those midwives and doctors who had been involved in the care of Know Your Midwife patients during all stages of childbirth felt that mothers benefitted from seeing the same midwife and getting to know her, doctors felt they 'wasted less time' seeing normal patients, midwives said that the midwives working within the scheme used their skills and they perceived them to have greater job satisfaction. When asked what their response would be if the present Know Your Midwife scheme were expanded to having more Teams, 31.5% of midwives felt that they would like to be included and the reasons they gave were: "I would expect better job satisfaction and utilisation of all my skills and an opportunity to follow through all parts of midwifery care. I would still want part time hours"; "Offers more scope to be a practitioner in one's own right."

When asked how they would respond if the Teams were expanded to include six midwives, 33.7% of midwives said that they would like to be included in such a Team and when asked if a domino scheme, similar to the Know Your Midwife scheme, but based in the community, were to be set up, 67.4% of midwives said that they would like to be involved in such a Team. Their reasons were "that greater job satisfaction would be achieved"; "This is how I see myself situated one day! Ideally involved with the woman and her family as a whole."

It is interesting that although in retrospect the Know Your Midwives appeared to have an exceedingly high workload (an average of 62.5 women to deliver per year each), a third of the midwives at St George's Hospital would have liked to have worked in the same way, as would have a third of the midwives had the Team been made into six (with a presumably lighter workload?). But had the scheme been based in the community and provided domino deliveries, two-thirds of the midwives working in the hospital would have liked to have taken part, which would appear to indicate that they perceived that the midwives in the Know Your Midwife scheme had increased job satisfaction and that they themselves perceived that they would have increased job satisfaction if they took part in such a scheme.

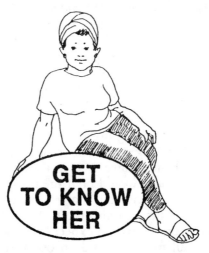

Social support in pregnancy outcome

In 1990 Ann Oakley, Linda Rajan and Adrian Grant, produced a paper in the *British Journal of Obstetrics and Gynaecology* detailing a study of 509 women with a history of low birth weight (previous babies being born of less than 2500 g). The study took place within four hospitals and women were randomised to receive either normal antenatal care (control group) or to receive normal standard antenatal care plus the intervention of a social support package by midwives, this consisted of a minimum of three home visits to be carried out at 14, 20 and 28 weeks of gestation, plus two telephone contacts or brief home visits during those times.

The midwives were also on call to the mothers for 24 hours a day and were supplied with radio pagers so that mothers could contact them. The research midwives gave advice or information about specific topics only if requested to do so by the mother and did not give any clinical care, for this they referred the women to either their GP, the Hospital or their Community Midwife. The intervention from the midwives giving social support appeared to have an effect on the 254 women who received it, compared to the 254 women in the control group. First, the babies were 38 g heavier than the control group babies and there were fewer very low birth weight babies in the group who had received social support from a midwife. Although the number of Hospital antenatal clinic visits was the same in both groups, more women in the control group were admitted to Hospital antenatally than women who were receiving social support from the midwife, both of which findings support the findings in the Know Your Midwife study. The women and babies who had received social support from midwives were significantly healthier in the early weeks following the births of their babies than those in the control group and women were very positive and appreciated the social support they had received. Eighty percent of those who had filled in the postnatal questionnaire singled out the fact that the midwife listened was very important to them.

Newcastle Community Midwifery Care Project

In 1987, Dr Frances Evans, Research Officer, wrote up her evaluation of a project. The aims of the project were:

1. To encourage the residents of Cowgate to use the Neighbourhood Centre for meeting their individual and group needs.
2. To develop a preventative community health and social work service.
3. To involve the various agencies, both statutory and voluntary, in cooperatively tackling the social problems of the Estates.
4. To provide Community-based midwifery care.
5. To promote the self-worth of the Community by involving people in the delivery of services.

This was a Community midwifery care project situated in the Cowgate and Newbiggin Hall Estates, two very deprived Council Estates in Newcastle upon Tyne. The project consisted of two pairs of midwives, one pair on each Estate, and they provided enhanced midwifery care to every mother in the project area. Women were visited in their homes at least four times during their pregnancy, a small number of the women were delivered by the project midwives and all the women were given postnatal care by the project midwives extended to 4 weeks postnatally with visits on the 14th, 21st and 28th day.

The Newbiggin Hall Team of Midwives worked from a Health Centre and in Cowgate the midwives were based in a Neighbourhood Centre. In the Cowgate Centre the midwives had an important role in the running and maintenance of the Neighbourhood Centre and there are distinct echoes of the Peckham Experiment reported by Innes Pearse (Pearse and Crocker, 1943; Pearse, 1979), one of the co-founders of the Pioneer Health Centre in Peckham which was founded in 1926 and was a holistic approach to health which consisted of care and refreshment to the whole community.

The midwifery intervention had an influence on outcome. There was a modification in the smoking and dietary habits of the women with enhanced midwifery intervention. The incidence of low birth weight babies was reduced and there was greater attendance at parentcraft classes by women who had enhanced midwifery visiting. Also the intervention reduced the incidence of preterm labour and reduced the use of pain relief during labour. But probably more important than any of these was that the scheme was incredibly popular with those women who received it.

Dr Evans' survey also shows that the midwives' job satisfaction levels were increased when they worked in this way:

> I have got a lot more job satisfaction. A lot more. Because you can read the benefits, you see the patients you have educated antenatally and they come out and they are able to cope. You can pick problems up because you have got the time to deal with them.

> We are able to give continuity of care. In hospital it is all interruptions, you sit down to help someone feed the baby and the phone rings, or it's the doctor's round, or the cleaner wants you, and it's all so fragmented. Somebody does all the babies,

somebody does all the fundal heights . . . with this, you go and see somebody and do everything that she needs and you finish with her before you move on to the next.

For me I think the highlight of the whole thing has been the dominos . . . getting to know somebody antenatally and actually delivering their baby, because I really enjoyed it, and then seeing them afterwards as well, it's an added bonus. The bond, it sounds sort of very romantic and everything, but the bond between the midwife and the woman who she delivers is really quite strong, and when you continue it through to the postnatal period it is much easier to look after them, and even still the bond now that I feel for the women I delivered is a lot stronger than with the other women I've looked after, so from their point of view it's much easier too.

Nottingham midwives in the 1950s

Julia Allison, who is now Head of Midwifery Studies at Norfolk College of Nursing and Midwifery, conducted a study of all the Community Midwives' registers from nearly 300 birth registers from retired District Midwives containing details of more than 35 000 home births from 1952 to 1966. Her study makes fascinating reading because although there is no evidence that there was continuity of care in this study, we know from the way that midwives worked at that time that total continuity of care was provided because the midwives had so little time off! Midwives frequently worked (and lived) together in pairs and one would be on duty when the other was off duty and vice versa. One of the most interesting facets of Allison's survey was of low birth weight babies by place of birth and neonatal death in Nottingham from 1952 to 1956.

Low birth weight babies by place of birth and neonatal death – Nottingham 1952–1966

	Born at home			Born in hospital		
Weight	*No. born*	*No. died*	*% died*	*No. born*	*No. died*	*% died*
Up to:						
3lb 4oz	115	66	57	641	455	71
4lb 6oz	268	37	14	937	162	17
4lb 15oz	378	20	5	931	70	8
5lb 8oz	1290	54	4	2026	91	5
Totals	2051	177	9	4535	778	17

Source: Allison, 1992.

Births, stillbirths and neonatal deaths in Nottingham by place of birth 1955–1972

	Total births (no.)		SB/neonatal deaths		SB/neonatal death rate	
Years	Home	Hospital	Home	Hospital	Home	Hospital
1955–1957	8011	7770	160	445	20.0	57.3
1958–1960	8672	8372	138	484	15.9	57.8
1961–1963	9354	9172	128	524	13.7	57.1
1964–1966	8062	10406	90	554	11.2	53.2
1967–1969	5987	11409	71	431	11.8	37.8
1970–1972	3682	11162	42	343	11.4	30.8
Total	43768	58291				

Source: Allison, 1992.

Category X clients

Jean Ball in her paper entitled 'Birthrate' describes the woman who appears to take up almost 30% of all admissions to the Labour Ward. These are the women who are basically 'false alarms', who do not need any further treatment and who are admitted unnecessarily for a period of anything from 1 hour to the Delivery Suite and more frequently are sent to the Antenatal Ward to await onset of labour. These are women who are having painful contractions or some other signs of labour but who are actually not in established labour.

Numbers of mothers in Category X (undelivered) shown as percentage of total cases (Trent Hospitals) over 3 months

Category X		% of all admissions
Unit	No.	
A	365	23.4
B	349	29.1
C	728	32.0
D	280	28.8
E	484	36.7
F	508	27.3
G	543	31.9
Total	3257	29.9

Estimated costs per hospital (based upon above data)

| Category X | | Costs per month | |
Unit	No.	£50	£120
A	121	6050	14520
B	116	5800	13920
C	243	12150	29160
D	93	4650	11160
E	161	8050	19230
F	169	8450	20280
G	181	9050	21720

Over a 3-month period Ball shows that in seven Trent hospitals the percentage of admissions who were Category X clients ranged from 23.4% of admissions to 36.7% of admissions to Labour Wards. She then goes on to give the estimated costs per hospital and says "that although it can be argued that much of the estimated costs arising come from fixed overheads such as heating and lighting, that reducing the number of admissions of Category X clients could save between £2000 and £14 000 per month and released midwife time to women who were actually in labour".

Although Category X clients can appear to be unrelated to continuity of care, if continuity of care schemes are drawn up in such a way as to reduce the number of Category X clients because women are assessed at home in early labour, the benefits which were seen from the Klein work described in Chapter 1 can be seen as part of such a system.

Michael Klein

In a comparative study of low-risk pregnant women 5005 births which took place in 1978 were studied. There was one intervention which appeared to have a significant effect upon women and that was when they were assessed in early labour at home by the Community Midwife or in their GP surgery by GP. This intervention appeared to lessen the need for induction of labour, epidural analgesia and forceps delivery. Women who were not offered this intervention appeared to have babies who

were often intubated and appeared to stay in hospital for longer
– 11 hours compared with 8 hours in hospital before the
delivery for primigravid women (the comparable duration in
multigravid women was 6 and 4 hours). The women who had
an assessment at home during early labour received less pethidine, they also received less fetal electronic monitoring, augmentation and their babies had less fetal distress. Thus it would
be recommended that when any system of maternity care is
going to be changed, one of the changes which could provide
most benefit to mothers and babies might be that of assessing
the woman in early labour at home rather than encouraging her
to come to hospital when she might be in false labour.

Job satisfaction

Before the Riverside Midwife Teams were set up in February
1989 a job satisfaction questionnaire was given to all midwifery
staff at both the Westminster Hospital, the West London
Hospital and the midwives working in the community. This
questionnaire was given out in June 1988, then again to the
midwifery staff now all working at the West London Hospital
or in the Community Teams in January 1990, and then again to
the midwives working in the Hospital Teams in the West
London Hospital and the Community Teams in May 1991.

The results are shown on pages 56 and 57.

Interpretation of the results

These 24 question questionnaires were given out prior to any
changes being made in 1988 (when there were two maternity
units and a community staff) in January–March 1990 when the
Community Teams had been set up and one of the Units (at the
Westminster Hospital) had been closed and the two Units
amalgamated. As can be seen for all the results, the job
satisfaction levels of the Community (Team) Midwives was
significantly higher than the job satisfaction levels of the
Hospital Midwives. * Indicates that the occurrence was 5 in

100 or less, which is unlikely to have been a chance result and means that the result is statistically significant; ** means that the occurrence was less than 1 in 100 which means that it is appreciably statistically significantly different; *** means that the occurrence was less than 1 in a 1000 which means that it is highly significantly different.

The results in May/June 1991 show a similarity of job satisfaction, the only statistically different result was in the amount of responsibility the midwives felt that they had in their present jobs. By this time the Hospital Midwives were working in Teams (albeit rather large teams), and although this had been hard to achieve this research shows that after the initiation of Hospital Teams the midwives found their job more satisfying than previously.

Cost savings of Riverside Community Teams in 1990

Total number of women looked after by Community Teams in 1990 = 646

Made up of home births = 42   hospital births = 604

Antenatal care by Community Teams costs £164 less than either GP or Hospital care (according to Harris, 1989)

Cost savings on 646 women = £105 944

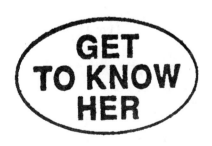

Results

	June–Oct. 1988 hospital	Jan.–March 1990 hospital

	June–Oct. 1988 hospital	Jan.–March 1990 hospital
Response rate to questionnaires	77 given out 50 (65%) returned	60 given out 31 (52%) returned
Sister Grade	29 of 50 (58%)	14 of 31 (45%)
Staff Midwife Grade	21 of 50 (42%)	17 of 31 (55%)
Average number of years having worked as a midwife	7¾ years	8½ years

Taking the job as a whole, how much job satisfaction does it provide you with?

A great deal	11 of 47 (23%)	9 of 31 (29%)
Quite a lot	23 of 37 (49%)	16 of 31 (52%)
A moderate amount	11 of 47 (23%)	5 of 31 (16%)
Very little	2 of 47 (4%)	1 of 31 (3%)

How often do you get a sense of achievement from your work?

Almost every day	33 of 44 (75%)	14 of 31 (45%)
About once a week	7 of 44 (16%)	12 of 31 (39%)
About every few weeks	4 of 44 (9%)	4 of 31 (13%)
Less than once a month	none	1 of 31 (3%)

Are your skills and knowledge fully used in your present job?

Yes	21 of 44 (48%)	13 of 27 (48%)
No	23 of 44 (52%)	14 of 27 (52%)

How much responsibility do you have in your present job?

A great deal	22 of 45 (49%)	10 of 31 (32%)
Quite a lot	19 of 45 (42%)	20 of 31 (65%)
Very little	4 of 45 (9%)	1 of 31 (3%)

How much responsibility would you like to have in your job?

More than now	24 of 45 (53%)	10 of 30 (33%)
Less than now	4 of 45 (9%)	none
About the same	17 of 45 (38%)	20 of 30 (66%)

Would you like to have the opportunity to take

More decisions than at present	36 of 43 (84%)	19 of 30 (63%)
Fewer decisions than now	none	none
Everything is fine as it is	7 of 43 (16%)	11 of 30 (37%)

Jan.–Mar. 1990 *Teams*	*May–June 1991* *hospital*	*May–June 1991* *Teams*

Jan.–Mar. 1990 *Teams*	*May–June 1991* *hospital*	*May–June 1991* *Teams*
24 given out 21 (87.5%) returned	60 given out 28 (47%) returned	25 given out 23 (92%) returned
21 of 21 (100%) none	14 of 28 (50%) 13 of 28 (46%)	23 of 23 (100%)
5⅓ years	7¼ years	5½ years
13 of 21 (62%) *** 6 of 21 (28%) 2 of 21 (10%) none	10 of 28 (36%) 11 of 28 (39%) 4 of 28 (14%) 2 of 28 (7%)	14 of 23 (61%) NS 8 of 23 (35%) 1 of 23 (4%) none
18 of 21 (86%) NS 2 of 21 (9%) 1 of 21 (5%) none	15 of 28 (54%) 10 of 28 (36%) 1 of 28 (4%) 1 of 28 (4%)	17 of 23 (74%) NS 5 of 23 (22%) 1 of 23 (4%) none
15 of 19 (79%) ** 4 of 19 (21%)	20 of 28 (71%) 6 of 28 (21%)	19 of 23 (83%) NS 3 of 23 (13%)
17 of 21 (81%) ** 3 of 21 (14%) 1 of 21 (5%)	10 of 28 (36%) 16 of 28 (57%) 2 of 28 (7%)	20 of 23 (87%)* 3 of 23 (13%) none
4 of 21 (19%) ** none 17 of 21 (81%) ***	12 of 28 (43%) none 16 of 28 (57%)	6 of 23 (26%) NS none 17 of 23 (74%) NS
8 of 21 (38%) *** none	13 of 28 (46%) none	12 of 23 (52%) NS none
13 of 21 (62%)	14 of 28 (50%)	11 of 23 (48%)

Labour Ward costs are the same, i.e.

	Hospital-based maternities:	Community-based maternities:
Spontaneous delivery rate	72%	72%
Caesarean deliveries	15%	15%
Episiotomies	24%	20%

Postnatal stay

	Hospital-based maternities:	Community-based maternities:
Average	3.43 days	3.0 days

Cost of postnatal stay = £300 per day
Cost of 0.43 of a day represents £129
for 604 women it represents £77 916

TOTAL COSTS SAVED BY COMMUNITY MIDWIFE TEAMS

Antenatal £105 944
Postnatal   £77 916

TOTAL £183 860

Extra costs of running this scheme = £55 000

ACTUAL COSTS SAVED £128 860

Cost savings appear to be achieved, women appear to be happier with continuity of carer, there appear to be no greater risks to women than with conventional care, midwives' job satisfaction appears to be enhanced – could it be that what women have been asking us for over the years might be better for midwives and the NHS too?

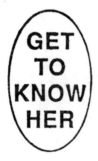
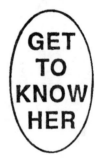

4

The named midwife — the ideal for the future?

Many of the schemes which have been described so far have tried to increase continuity of carer for women but the terms have been on the side of the midwives. Most schemes of this sort are those which are seen as feasible by midwives generally, but we should remember that women have never asked to be looked after by a team of midwives, they have always asked to be looked after by the same person all the way through their pregnancy, labour and puerperium.

Is there a way that we can provide individualised care, one midwife to one woman? Could this be at all practical? Perhaps we should do a few sums with present figures in mind.

Available hours of midwife time

At the moment each midwife works 37½ hours per week for 45 weeks per annum = 1687 hours per midwife per year.

In England and Wales there are 34 000 practising midwives (midwives who fill in an Intention to Practise form each year).

In England and Wales 740 000 women have babies each year.

Although 34 000 midwives fill in Intention to Practise forms each year it is obvious that not all of these midwives work in clinical practice, nor are all these midwives working full time. For a realistic estimate of the number of midwives who are actually doing 'hands on' clinical practice it would seem reasonable to subtract one-third of the total number of practising midwives and to work with a figure of two-thirds of the total:

⅔ of practising midwives is 22 666

Most women have approximately 12–14 antenatal visits taking approximately 12 hours of midwife time; the same is true of postnatal visits, these probably take up about 14 hours of midwife time. If we reckon that the average time a midwife needs to spend with a woman in labour is 14 hours we can then deduce that the average that each woman takes of midwife time is 40 hours. Add administration and travelling time, then each woman represents 45 hours of midwife time needed.

If the number of women giving birth each year is multiplied by the number of hours each woman needs of midwife time $740\,000 \times 40 = 33\,300\,000$ hours, we can see the number of midwife hours needed each year (not including hospital skeleton staff and intensive care for women having caesareans, etc.).

If we remember how many hours each midwife (whole-time equivalent) provides per year – 1687 (one midwife's hours per year) – the number of midwives needed to provide each woman in England and Wales with her own named midwife is 19 740 midwives each year.

Thus leaving 2926 midwives to act as skeleton staff in hospitals and to provide intensive care to mothers who need it.

For instance in a hospital delivering 4000 women per year the necessity would be for 111 midwives with caseloads of 36 women each plus a skeleton staff in the Labour Ward and Postnatal Ward of probably 28 midwives $(7 + 7 + 7 + 7)$. Total needed = 139 midwives.

In 1992 a Report on the Maternity Services was produced by an all party Select Committee. One of the recommendations was that midwives should have their own caseloads

> We recommend – that we should move as rapidly as possible towards a situation in which midwives have their own caseload and take full responsibility for the women who are under their care; (para 344)
> and that every woman should be able to get to know a midwife during the antenatal period who goes on to be with her in labour and then delivers her baby.
> We summarise the broad principles of our recommendations relating to maternity care as follows:
> — That the relationship between the woman and her care-givers is recognised as being of fundamental importance.
> — That schemes should be set up enabling women to get to know one or two health professionals during pregnancy who

will be with them during labour and delivery, whether at home or in hospital, and who will continue the care of mother and baby after birth. (para 384)

That same year (1992) the Patient's Charter Group issued a document called 'The Named Midwife', which was sent to all midwives, this pamphlet details the way in which 'The Named Midwife' concept could work.

A named qualified nurse, midwife or health visitor responsible for each patient. The Charter Standard is that you should have a named, qualified nurse, midwife or health visitor who will be reponsible for your nursing or midwifery care. ('The Named Midwife', p. 1)

In the United Kingdom there are over 100 000 qualified midwives – more than in any other country in the world. The fact that only 34 000 of them are actually registered as practising is in itself an extraordinary phenomenon that midwives, having spent a long time training and qualifying, do not go on to do the job for which they have trained. Training to be a midwife takes a not inconsiderable personal investment of time, energy and effort. The large drop-out rate may indicate a lack of satisfaction with the job as it is presently carried out in the NHS.

In 1990 the Institute of Manpower Studies carried out a study for the Royal College of Midwives on midwives' careers and grading (IMS Report No. 201) (Buchan and Stock, 1990). They were looking at what midwives found was most important in their job.

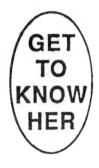

GET TO KNOW HER

Proportion indicating that each characteristic was in the three most important – by specialty

Characteristic	Hospital	Community	Total
Good career structure and prospects	35(3)	17	31
Attractive working environment	14	19	15
High professional status	12	14	12
Professionally rewarding client/ patient contact	64(1)	73(1)	66
Attractive remuneration	23	23	23
Manageable work load	22	22	22
Convenient working hours	20	17	19
Being able to use your initiative	29	50(2)	33
Availability of part-time work	19	7	16
Doing varied work	13	12	12
Making full use of professional skills	42(2)	41(3)	42
Other	0		0
Not answered	8	7	7
Total responses	100	100	100
N	553	138	691

Note: First, second and third ranking in brackets.
Source: IMS Table 7.4.

This table shows clearly that 'rewarding patient contact' is the most important facet of their job for both Community and Hospital Midwives. For Community Midwives the next most important part of their job was 'being able to use your initiative', whereas for Hospital Midwives the next most important factor was making full use of professional skills – the third most important factor for Community Midwives.

When both Hospital and Community Midwives were asked to look at the characteristics of each other's jobs they said: ·

Rating of NHS *Hospital Midwifery* by current status

Characteristic	Hospital Midwives	Community Midwives	Those not employed in NHS
Good career structure and prospects	35	36	32
Attractive working environment	31	14	20
High professional status	23	19	22
Professionally rewarding client/ patient contact	34	4	20
Attractive remuneration	12	13	8
Manageable work load	14	15	23
Convenient working hours	13	6	7
Being able to use your initiative	20	3	7
Availability of part-time work	41	19	34
Doing varied work	32	6	22
Making full use of professional skills	44	12	32
N	422	101	611

Source: IMS Table 7.5a.

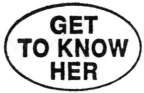

and

Rating of NHS *Community Midwifery* by current status

Characteristic	Hospital Midwives	Community Midwives	Those not employed in NHS
Good career structure and prospects	8	12	7
Attractive working environment	43	73	53
High professional status	18	33	23
Professionally rewarding client/ patient contact	57	92	65
Attractive remuneration	17	27	18
Manageable work load	26	19	24
Convenient working hours	18	21	13
Being able to use your initiative	53	74	58
Availability of part-time work	5	9	11
Doing varied work	21	46	29
Making full use of professional skills	41	70	50
N	422	115	111

Source: IMS Table 7.5b.

Thus Community Midwifery was seen by most midwives as being the most likely to provide midwives with the four most important characteristics for working:

1. Professionally rewarding client contact.
2. Making full use of professional skills.
3. Being able to use initiative.
4. Good career structure and prospects.

From this study it can be seen that the first consideration of midwives working in both hospital and the community is that of professionally rewarding client/patient contact – it is obvious from this study that midwives want to make a relationship with their clients in the same way that their clients want to make a relationship with them. The old adage 'Don't get involved' (Menzies, 1970) is obviously not appropriate for midwives. Midwives want to 'be friends' with women having babies, in the same way that women want to 'be friends' with their midwife.

The nature of the job – that it is of a limited duration, with a specific number of women – means that the friendship will not go on for ever (but with some women it might). It is a friendship of limited duration (9 months) and of varying intensity, quite shallow at first, rising to a crescendo during labour and very deep for the first few days after the birth, tailing off 4 weeks after the birth of the baby.

In the document 'Who's Left Holding the Baby?' (Nuffield Institute, 1992) one of the problems identified in modern maternity care is that midwives are seen as people who staff an area such as, the Antenatal Clinic, the Antenatal Ward, the Labour Ward or the Community, whereas what is really needed by women is a midwife to be where they are when they need them. Sometimes that is in their homes, and sometimes it is in the Hospital, sometimes in the Local Clinic, sometimes in the Ultrasound Department or the GP's surgery. If we try and leave the concept of staffing places or areas and go to the concept of staffing women, levels of staff might conceivably be changed and be much more flexible.

The Think Tank who wrote 'Who's left holding the baby?' suggests that if every midwife were to take on a caseload of between 24 and 38 women a year, the women's experience of the maternity services would radically alter and women would be enabled to have a named midwife and probably much happier childbirth experiences.

It is expected that each midwife who takes on (say) 36 women a year would work with another midwife so that they each have a caseload of 36 women, but that one of them would be available when the other was unavailable. It would be expected that these midwives would be on call all the time that they were working, but as they are not likely to be called more than once a week, for the 36 women they are looking after, this would be less arduous than it sounds.

If it could be envisaged that each of these midwives could also have considerable holiday, for instance, at the moment midwives work 37½ hours a week and, as we have seen, once the 5 weeks' holiday has been deducted plus ten Bank Holidays which is equivalent to seven working weeks, each midwife works an equivalent of 1687 hours per annum. As the midwife working in this way would work more intensely during working times the midwives could take 3 months' holiday. Thus one could have two midwives, we will call them Janet and Mary, Janet could decide that her holidays would be taken during the months of March, July and November, and Mary could decide that her holidays would be taken during the months of January, May and September.

Each of them would take on 36 women, who are due to deliver in the intervening months.

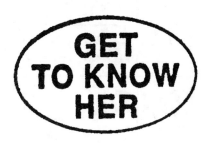

66

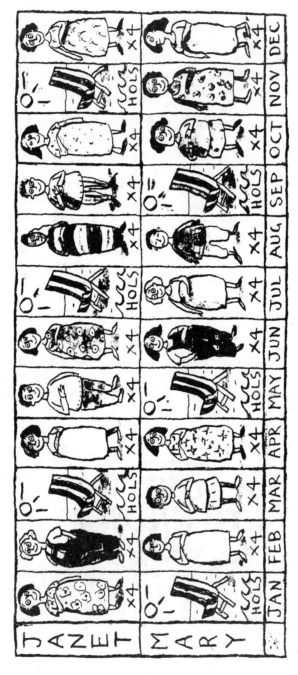

© Ant Parker

Janet and Mary will work out between them when they are going to have their holidays and if there is a particular month in their area which always seems to have a lot of babies (i.e. September, which is 9 months after Christmas), then neither of them would take a holiday during that month, and they would both be available.

If we look at how the scene would look during the month of April it is easy to see how it would appear to the midwives. The women who are due in November and December are not yet 12 weeks' pregnant, and would probably not have booked with the midwives. The women who are due in January, February and March would more or less have delivered and finished their postnatal care. So Janet would have 24 women that she is looking after at the moment (those from April, May, June, August, September and October) and Mary would have 20 women. Janet has a month's holiday in July to look forward to and Mary has a month's holiday in May and another month's holiday in September.

To be providing full care for 24 women is a feasible proposition for any midwife, each woman could be given the normal type of antenatal care in that particular area, so that she is seen regularly by her midwife throughout her pregnancy, she can also see her GP or an Obstetrician at an agreed number of visits, but she would be secure in the knowledge that she has a named midwife – who would carry a long range pager so that 'her' women had access to her whenever the woman needed her.

On going into labour a woman would bleep her midwife, who would go to the woman's home and assess the progress of her labour. This would eliminate what Jean Ball in 'Birthrate', has named Category X patients, who she estimates to be between 30% and 40% of any Labour Ward's admissions and who cost the maternity hospital up to £29 000 per month.

Category X patients are those women who go to the Labour Ward who think that they might be in labour, they are then assessed and are discovered not to be in established labour and they are then either sent home again or, more commonly, to the Antenatal Ward overnight with the cost implications of that action. Such women often have their labours induced just because they are there which has cost implications – inducing a labour which is not physiologically ready to start often leads to greater intervention at delivery, such as a caesarean section or forceps delivery with the cost implications of these actions.

With the named midwife assessing the woman in her own home the midwife would accompany the woman to hospital at the appropriate time, then deliver her baby (or the woman might deliver at home if that is what she wants). We have further evidence of the efficacy of women being assessed at home from the work of Klein published in 1983 (Klein *et al.*, 1983a,b) and mentioned in Chapter 1. Their study shows that when women who plan to deliver in hospital are assessed at home during early labour, several benefits accrue for them from the assessment at home:

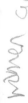

- They spend less time in hospital than a comparable group.
- They enter hospital in a more advanced stage of labour.
- They need less analgesia.
- They need less intervention.
- Their babies have less fetal distress.
- Their babies have higher Apgar scores.
- Their babies require less resuscitation.

All benefits gained by one small intervention – being assessed at home in early labour.

With this type of care women could deliver their babies at home or in hospital, they can be of low or high obstetric risk, it doesn't matter. Their need for obstetric input can be catered for in a flexible system in which their named midwife is with them when they need her, during labour, during a normal birth or during a caesarean section.

The midwives envisaged in this chapter are peripatetic, able to look after women in their homes or in hospital, and will have free and easy access to both the hospital and local facilities and will have full access to all investigations, both laboratory and ultrasound, they will be assumed to keep the GP notified of what they have arranged for the woman at all times, but they will not 'go through' the GP because of the ridiculous amount of time this takes. As is said in Para 219 of the Maternity Services Report:

We conclude that the desirable development of community-based antenatal care, combined with ready access to specialist assessment, will best be advanced by the general acceptance of the right of midwives to refer women directly to obstetricians or other appropriate specialists. Systems to ensure the prompt notification of GPs of such referrals will be necessary. (Para 243)

We recommend that protocols are drawn up in every District Health Authority and Health Board to ensure the rapid referral of babies becoming ill at home and requiring specialist attention. To facilitate this, the midwife should be able to refer directly to the paediatrician, while also notifying the GP of such referrals. (Para 344)

the right of midwives to admit women to NHS hospitals should be made explicit.

Students (both midwifery and medical) can easily be accommodated into this system, they are just linked to a midwife and they shadow her. In so doing they learn about midwifery, the progress of pregnancy, the different aspects of labour, the ups and downs of the puerperium, all with the same group of women – by seeing women all the way through students can learn more from them, hearing what they are saying, seeing what is happening to them, getting to know them, their other children, the circumstances in which they live. Human beings are eternally fascinating to other human beings, to practise fully as a midwife is like living in the most dramatic and fascinating soap opera – 'all human life is here' has never been more true.

The benefits of this type of education are detailed by Heseltine and Watkins (1991) as:

The student midwife is now able to recognise early in her training the practice of holistic care, and so develops into a more flexible and versatile practitioner.
Midwives, as part of their post-basic development, are undertaking research and surveys into other aspects of care.

The named midwife – how it could work in practice

It is becoming abundantly clear that the majority of midwives need to be peripatetic. They need to be where the woman needs them to be, sometimes it is in the woman's own home, sometimes it is a local health centre and sometimes it is in the hospital. For midwives to provide full care, i.e. a continuum of care throughout pregnancy, labour and delivery and the post-natal period to an individual woman, a midwife needs to be able to go to all the places where that woman is going to be.

One can imagine that a woman might start her pregnancy by going to a local midwives' clinic, perhaps based in a GP's surgery, for pregnancy testing or for early pregnancy counsel-ling. When the date of her last menstrual period is ascertained and the likely date that her baby is due, a midwife could be allocated to her, who then remains her midwife through thick and thin, whatever happens to that woman, whether she miscarries at 11 weeks, whether she develops diabetes in pregnancy at 32 weeks, whether she needs a caesarean section at 41 weeks or whether she progresses normally at home or in hospital. The main concept has to be that the woman and the midwife are bonded together and accompany each other at each aspect of that care.

The lead professional

It may be a midwife who provides all the antenatal, labour and delivery and postnatal care for a woman, on the other hand it could be a GP or an Obstetrician, but as both GPs and Obstetricians find it difficult to provide the whole gamut of care they may find that they need to work with a midwife or midwives to provide the whole gamut of care, and working in this way could be an option for those midwives who find it difficult to commit themselves to being on call and who wish to work part-time or who are unable to be flexible in the hours that they work.

Whoever takes on the role of 'lead professional' for that particular woman, be it midwife or doctor, the woman needs to know that her lead professional will be with her through thick and thin and especially when the woman needs the lead professional most – when she is in pain and when she is getting tired and fed up.

When a woman has a midwife who is 'her lead professional' or, in other words, 'her midwife' she has access to that midwife 24 hours a day, and can bleep her to discuss different aspects of the pregnancy whenever she needs to. As has been suggested in another chapter it is a good idea to get women trained so that more easily than if they are delivered with force into a hard, noisy environment. There is very little evidence to support this but there was an interesting article (Jacobson *et al.*, 1987) on the 'Perinatal origin of adult self-destructive behaviour' published in the *Scandinavian Journal of Psychiatry* in 1987 which describes a study of the birth records of 412 victims of suicide, alcoholism and drug addiction, who were born in Stockholm after 1940 and who died there between 1978 and 1984, compared to 2901 controls. The birth records of the 412 suicide victims showed that suicides involving asphyxiation were closely associated with asphyxia at birth. Suicides by violent mechanical means such as by hanging or from leaping off a bridge or high building, were associated with mechanical birth trauma, and drug addiction was associated with opiate and/or barbiturate administration to mothers during labour. The Study suggests that obstetric procedures should be carefully evaluated and possibly modified to prevent eventual self-destructive behaviour.

By enabling the woman to have a 'friend on the inside' – her own midwife, her named midwife, a midwife with her own caseload which includes this woman – then it is almost guaranteed that women will be treated more gently and with greater sensitivity – it is difficult to be unkind to your friend after all.

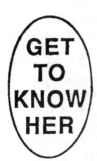

they not only leave their phone number, but a comprehensive message when they bleep the midwife so that she knows whether it is necessary to drop everything and return the call immediately or whether it can wait until tomorrow.

The midwife can carry out antenatal care on the woman in a Local Health Authority Clinic, GP's Surgery, Hospital Antenatal Clinic or in the woman's home. The midwife needs to arrange the venue that is most convenient for the woman and for herself. The woman might see her GP for a heart and lung examination at some time during the pregnancy. She might see a Consultant Obstetrician at 28 weeks or 36 weeks or at another time arranged between the mother, midwife and the Obstetrician. For antenatal care the midwife can use the time-honoured routine of every 4 weeks until 28 weeks, every 2 weeks until 36 weeks and every week until labour, or she might consider using the schedule approved by the Royal College of Obstetricians and Gynaecologists and suggested by Marion Hall, an Obstetrician from Aberdeen, who showed that the great number of visits that women are subjected to have no basis of research evidence to recommend them.

In the report of the Royal College of Obstetricians and Gynaecologists Working Party on Antenatal and Intrapartum Care 1982, published by the Royal College of Obstetricians and Gynaecologists, the following is suggested:

Suggestions for shared antenatal care:

1. It is thought that in the normal low-risk case a minimum of five visits is required. These must be done by a combination of Specialist Obstetrician, GP and midwife. They should be at 12, 20, 28–32, 36 weeks and term. A special visit for alphafetoprotein (AFP) screening may be required at 16–18 weeks, but the woman would not require a full examination at that time.
2. The amount of antenatal care will vary depending on circumstances but the following format is suggested, based on the work of Hall *et al.* (1980):

At 12 weeks   – the pregnant woman is – Obstetrician booked for care and confinement and determination of gestation

At 16–18 weeks	– for alphafetoprotein screening and other blood tests	– GP/midwife
At 22 weeks	– for baseline weight for IUGR prediction	– GP/midwife
At 26 weeks	– primigravidae only	– GP/midwife
At 30 weeks	– for selection for IUGR and pregnancy-induced hypertension screening	– Obstetrician
At 34 weeks	– primigravidae only	– GP/midwife
At 36 weeks	– for detection of malpresentation and PIH screening	– GP/midwife
At 38 weeks	– primigravidae only	– GP/midwife
At 40 weeks	– for assessment of delivery	– Obstetrician

On the other hand in *Pregnancy and Risk – The Basis for Rational Management* Professor Gordon Stirrat in his chapter states:

Patterns of care are presently under scrutiny. The traditional scheme of visits, every 4 weeks until 28, every 2 weeks from 28 to 36 and weekly thereafter, has not been proved necessary in women at low risk of developing complications. It has been suggested that, in the absence of complications, the patient should be seen by a midwife and/or doctor at:
● 12 weeks – to arrange booking and confirm dates.
● 16 weeks – baseline weight and blood pressure: screening tests (e.g. ultrasound, AFP).
● 26 weeks – to check fetal growth.
● 36 weeks – to check presentation.
● 40 weeks – assessment near delivery.

Any additional visits should have a clearly specified objective.

The midwife may decide that she will carry out the number o: visits in either of these schedules, and as evidence is collected i: is exceedingly unlikely that in the future so many women wil see an Obstetrician or GP, except for specific medical reasons The basis of this statement comes from the evidence ir Chalmers *et al.* (1989), *Effective Care in Pregnancy and Child-birth*:

Appendix 4 – Forms of care that should be abandoned in the light of the available evidence
Involving doctors in the care of all women during pregnancy,
Involving obstetricians in the care of all women during pregnancy,
Insisting on universal institutional confinement.
As technical advances became more complex, care has come to be increasingly controlled by, if not carried out by specialist obstetricians. The benefits of this trend can be seriously challenged. It is inherently unwise, and perhaps unsafe, for women with normal pregnancies to be cared for by obstetric specialists, even if the required personnel were available. Specialists caring for women with both normal and abnormal pregnancies, because of time constraints, have to make an impossible choice: to neglect the normal pregnancies in order to concentrate their care on those with pathology, or to spend most of their tim supervising biologically normal processes, in which case the would rapidly lose their specialist expertise. Midwives an general practitioners, on the other hand, are primarily orient to the care of women with normal pregnancies, and are likely have more detailed knowledge of the particular circumstances individual women. The care that they can give to the majority women whose pregnancies are not affected by any major ill or serious complication will often be more responsive to t needs than that given by specialist obstetricians.

The chapter then continues with a plea for coop between the three specialties and a putting away of the that have been inherent between the professions inv childbirth for so long.

Does it really matter how babies are born?

Some midwives feel that if babies are born gentl respect and love they will be likely to cope with lif(

5

Examples of continuity of carer. Domino deliveries

Domino deliveries have for many years been seen as the answer to women's desire to have continuity of carer combined with a hospital delivery and of coming home very soon following the delivery. In fact domino deliveries have really been nothing more or less than a confidence trick for most women. According to statistics collected by the Department of Health and shown by Macfarlane and Mugford (1984) in charts in 'Birth Counts' published by HMSO, the number of women having a domino system has never been greater than 4% (1985) and by 1987–88 had fallen to 3.5% of women, and these statistics also included women delivered in GP Units by Community Midwives. Savage is quoted in *Pregnancy Care in the 1990s*:

> The major problem which faces midwives in the educational field is the limited number of home deliveries, that is, 1%, only half of which are planned, Domino deliveries (3%) and GP Unit deliveries (7%) available for teaching midwifery students about primary intrapartum maternity care. (Chamberlain and Zander, 1992, p. 72)

The more sinister factor when the number of women having domino deliveries is almost as low as for women having home births is that women have known for many years that it is almost impossible to obtain a home birth, but many women have believed – and been led to believe – that it is perfectly feasible to have a domino delivery; when in fact it has actually been almost impossible to obtain a domino delivery as well.

Domino deliveries have been promoted by government sources and by the Royal College of Obstetricians and Gynaecologists – in the 'Pregnancy Book', published by the Health Education Authority, it says:

THE DOMINO SYSTEM
'Domino' is a shortening of 'Domiciliary-In-Out'. Under this system you are mainly looked after by your community midwife, mostly at home – which is called domiciliary care. She will get to know you before the birth, take you into hospital when you go into labour, and deliver your baby. (Your GP or the hospital doctor will be available to help if they are needed.) If you and your baby are well, you can go home early (say, in six hours) and your midwife continues to look after you at home. So the advantage of this system is that one person is usually able to care for you right the way through. You can get to know each other well.

Pregnancy dated Autumn/Winter 1989–90 says:

THE DOMINO SYSTEM
Domino actually means 'Domiciliary-In-Out' and is similar to a birth in a GP unit. A community midwife is responsible for your antenatal care, visits you at home and takes you into hospital to deliver your baby when you go into labour. If all goes well you can be home within six hours and your midwife will carry on looking after you there – many mums who opt for this system come to regard her as a friend for life.

By its Spring/Summer 1990 issue *Pregnancy* had changed the emphasis of its words so that they are more realistic:

THE DOMINO SYSTEM
Standing for 'Domiciliary-In-Out', this is similar to birth in a GP unit. Throughout your pregnancy you will be looked after by a community midwife who will visit you at home, then take you into hospital when you go into labour and deliver you herself. If all goes well you can be home within six hours where the midwife will continue looking after you. Advantages are that you will have built up a rapport with the midwife during your pregnancy, *though there is a possibility she won't be around to deliver you and you may end up being supervised by a stranger.* A variation of the domino system is when you see several midwives during your pregnancy, one of whom will be present at birth. *The term 'domino system' is sometimes used loosely by hospital, meaning simply a short stay with the birth overseen by a hospital midwife,* so do check.

In *Mother & Baby* July 1990 issue there is an attractive chart:

DOMINO

```
ANTENATAL CARE
By your GP and midwife at the
surgery or at home
```

```
BIRTH
Your midwife looks after you at
home during early labour and
takes you to the hospital or GP
unit just for the birth. You are
taken home after a few hours
```

Many women are exceedingly disappointed that when they book for a domino delivery, first, it is quite difficult to get to know a Community Midwife and, secondly, if a woman does get to know a Community Midwife, the likelihood of 'her' Community Midwife actually attending in labour is remote. She may be busy, otherwise engaged, off duty, on holiday or generally not available. In many areas even if the Community Midwife is available and willing to look after the woman in labour, local policy decrees that she must not come into the labour ward and look after a woman when she is not on call – if she does she will either, not get paid for the time she spends there, or she will be criticised for thinking that she is 'indispensible' and for not leaving the woman to her colleagues – "do you think you are better than the midwives in the labour ward?" – as long as we see this for what it is, the nursing philosophy of 'not getting involved' described by Isobel Menzies (1970), which has no place in nursing and even less relevance in midwifery.

For many women their midwife's suggestion will be that they should go into hospital to be assessed by the midwives in the Hospital Labour Ward. Once this happens as the Hospital Midwife and the women have been working together for some time the Community Midwife does not come in, but the Hospital Midwife stays with the woman in labour until the end of her shift when another midwife comes, so that continuity of care is not achieved nor is there any difference in the sort of care the woman receives from any other woman booking for hospital care.

In retrospect, if the woman has been happy with her Hospital Midwives (which, it has to be said, they invariably are), this whole scenario may not appear significant, but if a woman has been planning and has specifically tried to achieve a domino delivery, and she is then fobbed off with a normal hospital birth with a Hospital Midwife and no attempts are made for her to have continuity of carer, it can indeed be a great disappointment to her.

When setting up Team Schemes, domino deliveries can be incorporated as part of the whole system. As was the case in the Know Your Midwife Scheme at St George's in Tooting, South London, although the midwives in this scheme were hospital based, they were peripatetic and cared for the women wherever the women needed them to be for the first 18 months of the trial. Similar schemes are taking place in Riverside Health Authority, Oxford, Harlow New Town and Oxford.

With the Know Your Midwife Team although the Team was hospital based, they did some antenatal care at home (for those pregnant women who found it hard to get to the Antenatal Clinic), they did postnatal care at home and for the first 18 months of the project they visited women in early labour at home, but after 18 months of the trial this was stopped by the Director of Midwifery Services for no given reason. Most of the results were therefore of women who had been assessed at home in early labour.

Let us look in depth at some of these schemes, those which provide most successful continuity of carer are invariably based in the community, some of the schemes are based in hospital but are at the same time peripatetic such as:

The Know Your Midwife scheme at St George's, Tooting

Between April 1983 and August 1985, 503 women were looked after throughout their pregnancy, labour and puerperium by a Team of four midwives called the 'Know Your Midwife Team' (KYM). So that the effects of this type of care could be scientifically evaluated a randomised controlled trial was set up. In the trial were 1001 pregnant women deemed to be at low obstetric risk. The definition of 'low risk' was that all women included must fall within the following criteria:

- Over 5 feet tall.
- No serious medical problems.
- No previous uterine surgery.
- No more than two miscarriages or terminations of pregnancy.
- No previous stillborn babies or neonatal deaths.
- No previous intrauterine growth retardation.
- No previous preterm labours.
- No rhesus antibodies.

Forty-three of the women offered KYM care refused it and had the same care as the Control Group, but consistent with the theory of randomisation, their results were kept in the original group to which they had been allocated.

The groups were compared in terms of feasibility, patient satisfaction, obstetric outcome and cost.

The women came to the normal Booking Clinic at St George's Hospital, Tooting, where they were interviewed by a midwife who took a full medical and social history, and they were then examined by an Obstetrician. The Obstetrician in whose name the woman was booked, or one of his team, saw the woman at the Booking Clinic, at a routine visit at 36 weeks of pregnancy, and again if the pregnancy lasted over 41 weeks. If the midwives ever felt that it was necessary to refer a woman to a doctor, a member of the Obstetric Staff was asked to see the woman or her baby.

Following the Booking Clinic women who fell into the criteria listed above had sealed opaque envelopes clipped to their notes and inside the envelopes was the legend KYM or the

Antenatal care

A pilot scheme for antenatal services in South London has been set up as a result of recommendations in the Short Report. Reva Klein visited the scheme which provides continuity of care to 240 mothers-to-be

Mothering instincts

AN EXCITING pilot scheme at St George's Hospital in South London is designed to take the doldrums out of maternity care — for both mothers and midwives. The midwifery project aims to give women individualised continuity of care not normally known outside the district midwifery services. And it allows the midwives to take responsibility and make use of their skills in the fullest sense.

The scheme involves four midwives caring for 240 women a year. The midwives work on a 24-hour rota, but can choose to see a woman through labour after her shift finishes, if both parties wish. Women are seen by the consultant only twice during their pregnancy, if there are no complications; at their first antenatal visit, and at 36 weeks. The remainder of the time, all examinations and tests are carried out by the four midwives, who will also be on call to explain and talk over things after consultations with doctors. All women are given the opportunity to speak to health visitors and social workers and a psychologist if they want to, on an informal basis.

Despite the radical nature of the project, there has been little in the way of obstacles. The idea behind it owes much to the Short Report of 1980, which looked at how the skills of midwives were being utilised, how women were being cared for, and made recommendations on ways of facilitating improvements in the maternity services. Lynne Murray, director of midwifery services at St George's and the beleaguered South London Hospital for Women, set up a working party to look at specific aspects of the report. She was part of a multi-disciplinary team examining their antenatal department. 'We looked to see whether we were fulfilling the recommendations of the report and if not, how we could' she said.

The answer, after clearance by the district nursing officer, was the setting up of the midwifery project. The scheme had to be passed by the Nursing Ethical Committee, and the three consultants and a professor were consulted and agreed to hand over some of their cases to the midwives. So far, the district is financing the project through the normal midwifery budget, but it is hoped that funding will be contributed by the regional budget. 'If we can get outside money,' says Mrs Murray, 'we would be able to afford extras, like bleeps and a research assistant.' In the meantime, a committee is being set up to evaluate the project.

Caroline Flint, the midwifery sister directly responsible for the project, believes it will prove to be an economic way of using skilled staff. 'This is a huge commitment in terms of time and finance on the part of midwifery management. We're taking four people out of the general service to run the project. But in the long run, it will be cheaper because you'll have a midwife there when needed who won't be paid when it's not necessary for her to be there. Our system is along the lines of the district midwifery service, working in small teams.'

A keynote of the project is accessibility. Women coming in to the clinic get to know the midwives personally over a period of time, and know that they can talk to them about any worries they may have, no matter how 'trivial.' In addition, Sister Flint holds weekly Friday morning sessions, during which time women can come in and talk about any problems or worries they may have. There is one evening clinic a week for working mothers which is, unsurprisingly overwhelmingly popular.

It is altogether a friendly clinic, for both those in the project and those not. Women are relaxed, sit and chat, have the use of adjacent creche for toddlers in tow and can watch health education video films, run on a regular basis. Live teaching aids are another feature: a recently delivered mother will come to talk about her experiences of giving birth at the hospital, or a psychologist will talk about child development, while women are in the waiting area. At the moment, women go to standard antenatal classes held at the hospital, but Sister Flint envisages conducting the classes more informally, while the women are waiting to be seen.

Although consultants' beds and labour rooms are used, and the obstetricians are on 24-hour call, there is a great deal of flexibility in terms of labour and delivery. As Sister Flint puts it: 'Because we have six months in which to get to know the women so well, we get to know what they want and what their expectations and fears are concerning labour and delivery.' There is a place in everyone's notes for stating specific requests, do's and don'ts. The labour room itself is fitted out with mats birthing chairs and a bean-bag to enable women to make themselves as comfortable as they choose. And it goes without saying that individuals' rights of choice are respected.

After a few years, Mrs Murray says she would like to see the programme expand so that it could be offered to more women, with more midwives taking part And the expansion need not be confined to merely numbers. As Sister Flint points out: 'Women in the high risk category need continuity of care, too — perhaps even more than low risk women. This concept can be developed further, in time.'   □

slip of paper said CONTROL. Thus 503 women were randomised into the KYM Group and 498 into the Control Group.

How did it work for the women?

The women came to St George's Hospital in Tooting and were booked through the normal Booking Clinic, which consisted of an interview with a midwife, a physical examination by a doctor, and blood being taken and an appointment being made for an ultrasound scan. The woman was asked many questions about her physical, medical and emotional health, and this was all put in her hospital notes.

If the woman had been randomised into the group receiving care from the KYM Team she received a letter within the next few days, inviting her to take part in the KYM Scheme. The letter described the way the scheme worked and she was given a change of appointment if she wished to become part of the KYM Scheme. The change of appointment was for an appointment at the KYM Clinic rather than the normal Hospital Clinic that she was expecting to come to.

Women receiving care from the KYM Team came to clinics on any day of the week. There were small clinics on Monday, Tuesday, Thursday and Friday when women were seen at half hour intervals at 2 p.m., 2.30 p.m., 3 p.m., 3.30 p.m. and 4 p.m. There was a much larger clinic on a Wednesday which carried on into the evening. Women were seen from 1 p.m. until 9 p.m., but there was a break between 4.30 p.m. and 6 p.m. when no appointments were made and the Know Your Midwives had their weekly meeting to develop their relationship with each other, to compare and share clinical experiences, to discuss their clients and any problems that were cropping up and to formulate policy for the future. An example of the Know Your Midwives off duty can be seen in Chapter 7.

For the midwives there were two duty spans except for Wednesdays. The early shift entailed coming on duty at 8 a.m., visiting all the women in the postnatal wards who had been delivered in the scheme (usually about four to five women), providing their postnatal checks and giving breastfeeding advice and the usual type of care that postnatal women need. Then the midwife would go to the antenatal ward to liaise with any women in the antenatal ward and then she would go out into the community to carry out postnatal care on women from the scheme who had been delivered and discharged (this was usually about four to five women). At lunch time this same midwife would come back into the hospital and from 2 p.m. she would see five pregnant women in the Antenatal Clinic. The other duty was being on call; the midwife was on call for 24 hours from 7.45 a.m. to 7.45 a.m. the following morning. She was not expected to do anything but stay at home and wait to be bleeped. In the evening she was expected to do postnatal care on any women on the Scheme who needed this, so she would go into the hospital and carry out postnatal care on the women in the hospital and would expect to go home from the hospital between 7 and 8 p.m. The Know Your Midwife on call responded to any calls on the bleeper. On a Wednesday one of the midwives worked from 1 p.m. until 9 p.m. and in that time she did nothing else but antenatal care. Because the early shift midwife was also in the Antenatal Clinic on Wednesday afternoon there were two midwives doing antenatal care on their clients during this time. Wednesday was chosen as the day on which to hold the big Antenatal Clinic because one of the Consultant Obstetricians also had his clinic on this day and he was very good at turning breeches – this skill proved very useful for several women whose babies were presenting in the breech position.

The women were seen by all four Know Your Midwives in the antenatal period. When they went into labour they bleeped the Team and the bleep was responded to by the midwife on call. For the first 18 months of the Scheme the on call midwife would go to the woman's home and assess her in early labour. This was then stopped by a decree from the Director of Midwifery Services and the Professor of Obstetrics and the midwife had to assess the woman in hospital which involved a greater time commitment and was therefore less efficient.

The women were looked after by a midwife they knew throughout their labour and were delivered in the St George's Labour Ward by one of the Know Your Midwives. After their baby was born the women usually went to the Postnatal Ward for a varying length of time. Some stayed for 1 day, some stayed for 4 or 5, very few of the women went home immediately after delivery, but if they wanted to they could.

The women were followed up at 6 weeks following delivery. The benefits of KYM care were seen in greater confidence of the women who had received that care and a more positive attitude to the experience they had been through compared with the Control Group who had received normal hospital care.

The other midwives

In Chapter 3 the research project carried out by the Director of Midwifery Services is described, and it can be seen that many of the midwives within the hospital were very enthusiastic at the thought of joining a similar Scheme to the KYM Scheme, and even more enthusiastic about joining a similar Scheme based in the Community with women being able to get to know their midwife and having domino deliveries.

Each of the midwives who took part in the KYM Scheme was asked to give her comments on her time spent in the Scheme. Wendy Pearce wrote a diary of a 24 hour day during which time she delivers two babies which was published in the Know Your Midwife Report. In *Nursing Times* (30 January 1985) Claire Neil says:

> for the first time since working as a midwife I have the support of a closely knit team and I am able to confide experiences and discuss difficulties. This change in the way I am now working has helped me to develop more knowledge. The Scheme has helped me to re-establish confidence in my midwifery skills because every aspect of these skills is being called into use by the way I am working.
>
> Working in this way offering continuity of care has formed reciprocal benefits for both the mother and for me as a practising midwife. I have the strong impression that being able to offer continuity of care restores the meaning of a midwife, enhancing immeasurably the benefits for the childbearing woman and her baby. (Neil, 1985).

Penny Church says:

> working closely together has enabled us to learn from one another and being able to talk things through openly and honestly without feeling threatened, has provided a stimulating

environment for discussion and learning development. The feedback from the women we have been caring for has been very positive, indicating that they have enjoyed being involved in the Scheme. This positive feedback has made the long hours we occasionally work, very worthwhile.

April Gloag's words were:

> I felt the care the mothers and babies received was excellent. The comments I heard from many mothers was that they really enjoyed being treated as individuals, that they felt they received a lot of support from the KYM team throughout their pregnancy, delivery and puerperium, the fact that they could lift up a telephone and contact a midwife that they knew at any time of the day or night they found very reassuring, and the fact that they knew that one of the team of four would be delivering them took a great deal of fear out of that situation.

Clover Dixon joined the Scheme towards the end of the research period, she said:

> When a lady went into labour she was reassured because she knew that the midwife who would be with her in labour and would deliver her would be a midwife she knew. One lady told me how pleasant it was to be greeted by her midwife by her first name when she was feeling frightened of the unknown – it was a lovely beginning to an unforgettable and rewarding experience. As a midwife I gained in confidence by seeing women all the way through.

The research project

Feasibility

In order to ascertain whether the women on the KYM Scheme were actually seeing less care-givers an in-depth study of those 101 women booked to deliver in September and October 1984 was undertaken. This was to ascertain who each woman saw at each antenatal visit and who she had with her during labour, whether there was any difference in the number of care-givers the two Groups saw and whether they had someone with them during labour who they had been able to get to know during their pregnancy.

The women's satisfaction

In order to measure client satisfaction, three questionnaires were used. These were given out at 37 weeks of pregnancy, 2 days following delivery and 6 weeks following delivery when they were accompanied by a General Health Questionnaire. The Questionnaires were always given out and collected by the Research Assistant or the Secretary and not by the midwives, in order to avoid bias. Women in the hospital were receiving Questionnaires if they were in the KYM Group, in the Control Group or if they were having Shared Care because the researchers were conducting a parallel study into women receiving shared care from their GPs, so the general opinion seemed to be that it was a normal part of pregnancy and early parenthood in that hospital to receive Questionnaires.

Obstetric outcome

The obstetric data sheet was filled in from the notes of every woman in the Study, this included all details of length of pregnancy, antenatal admissions, initiation of labour, analgesia used during labour, length of labour, type of delivery, perineal trauma, estimated blood loss, haemoglobin levels at 36 weeks and 2 days postnatally and details of the baby.

Cost

There were some consequences of the differing types of care which had obvious cost implications and these were compared. The cost of antenatal admissions was lower in the KYM Group as they had less admissions, the women in the Research Group also had less epidurals during labour, there were cost implications in this.

It was estimated that the cost of epidurals for the KYM Group (88 had epidurals) was approximately £19 360 over the 2-year period and the cost of epidurals for the Control Group (143 had epidurals) was approximately £31 460, representing a cost saving of £12 100 in 500 women, not a huge amount but when extrapolated to the 740 000 women every year who give birth in the UK the results are staggering.

17.2% (80) of women in the KYM Group compared with 24.9% (114) of women in the Control Group had their labours accelerated, this had cost implications considering that at the time the cost of acceleration of labour per client in a Midlands Hospital was estimated to be £11.44p. Only £388.96 was saved in this instance, but had the scheme been carried out with more women the savings would have been correspondingly greater.

£24.800 was estimated to have been saved by the KYM Scheme in savings on antenatal admissions. The KYM women spent a total of 920 days on an Antenatal Ward compared with 1075 for the Control Group. Antenatal care also cost less for the KYM Group as is described later.

The two randomised Groups were similar in terms of parity, age and socioeconomic class, there was a racial difference in that there were less Asian women in the KYM Group than in the Control Group (9.5% compared with 18.2%), but the numbers of European and Afro-caribbean women were similar. In any findings which were likely to be affected by this, race was controlled for.

The research showed that the women looked after by the KYM midwives saw less care-givers antenatally and they normally had someone with them in labour whom they had been able to get to know during their pregnancy, they were more satisfied with their antenatal care, they felt more prepared for labour and for motherhood, they felt more in control during labour and they found labour a more positive experience than did the Control Group. Both groups found midwives more approachable than doctors during the antenatal period.

During labour women in the KYM Group had longer first stages of labour, but less analgesia and more chance of a normal delivery.

The study showed that midwife care cost less than conventional care, not only because midwives are paid less than medical personnel, but because the type of care they give has less cost implications. Women in the KYM Group had less antenatal admissions and less epidurals – both having significant cost implications.

When women were seen in the Antenatal Clinic, KYM women only saw a midwife, whereas women in the Control Group saw a receptionist, someone who tested their urine, a

Doctor plus a midwife or nurse who would be assisting. It was estimated that antenatal care costs for the Control Group were 25% more than costs of antenatal care for KYM women.

The Women's satisfaction

	KYM	Control	
Being able to discuss anxieties easily in Clinic	89.3% (243)	76.6% (200)	***
Midwives very helpful with anxieties	83.7% (220)	55.3% (140)	***
Doctors very helpful with anxieties	33.9% (75)	38.5% (95)	NS
Satisfied with Antenatal Clinic	94.5% (259)	86.8% (230)	**
Labour (questions answered at 2 days postnatal)			
Felt very well prepared	52.4% (144)	40.2% (102)	**
Able to choose position in labour all of the time	53.1% (139)	33.1% (83)	***
At 6 weeks postnatally			
Wonderful/enjoyable labour	42.3% (104)	32.2% (72)	*
Very much in control during labour	41.9% (103)	24.0% (96)	***
All choices in labour always explained	61.1% (149)	38.4% (86)	***
Very satisfied with pain relief	57.9% (121)	50.7% (104)	NS
Very well prepared for looking after a baby	43.0% (104)	28.8% (64)	***
Easy being a mother	19.8% (49)	10.2% (23)	*

* P<0.05.
** P<0.01.
***P<0.001.
( ) indicates numbers.
Source: Flint and Poulengeris, 1987.

Obstetric outcome

	KYM	Control	
Pregnancy lasting 37–41 weeks	89.8%	89.6%	NS
Total days of antenatal admission	920	1075	NS
Spontaneous onset of labour	71.8%	62.0%	**
Accelerated labour	17.2%	24.9%	**
Induced labour	11.0%	13.1%	**
Artificial rupture of membranes	53.1%	59.5%	NS
Mean length of first stage of labour (primips)	9 hrs 30 mins	7 hrs 47 mins	**
No analgesia or only Entonox	51.4%	38.1%	***
Epidural	18.3%	30.2%	***
Normal delivery in primips	69.7%	61.8%	NS
Instrumental delivery in primigravidae	19.3%	28.0%	NS
Caesarean section in primigravidae	10.9%	10.2%	NS
Episiotomy in primigravidae	46.5%	62.3%	***
Live baby	96.3%	97.5%	
Stillborn baby	0.8%	0.4%	
Died in first month	0.8%	0.4%	
Mean birthweight	3.284 kg	3.218 kg	NS

Apgar score at 1 minute 8 and above	80.9%	80.5%	NS
Apgar score at 5 minutes 8 and above	96.4%	98.7%	*
Admission to SCBU	4.8%	4.5%	NS

*   P<0.05.
** P<0.01.
***P<0.001.
Source: Flint and Poulengeris, 1987.

As can be seen from the figures in the tables above from the KYM Scheme, many benefits ensued from being able to get to know a small group of midwives who guaranteed to look after them throughout their pregnancy, labour and puerperium. Women were more able to discuss their anxieties antenatally, they found the midwives exceedingly helpful with anxieties, they were satisfied with their antenatal care, they felt very well prepared for labour, they were able to choose a comfortable position in labour all of the time. Six weeks after they had had their babies they looked back on their labour as a wonderful or enjoyable experience of which they felt very much in control. They also felt all their choices had been explained to them. They felt very well prepared for looking after a baby and they found it easier being a mother than did the women in the Control Group.

Interestingly, both groups were equally satisfied with pain relief despite the fact that the KYM Group had had far less pain relief than the control group. The scheme had obvious benefits for women but also apparently for midwives. The scheme was greatly harmed in December 1984, when one of the midwives was disciplined for specious reasons. In retrospect it can be seen that this sabotage was mainly prompted by professional jealousy and from that moment the Scheme limped on for a further few months and was stopped at the end of the 2-year period, the reason given was for an evaluation to take place.

Following the highly successful evaluation, the KYM Scheme has never been reinstated, but this is not surprising. The enormous energy and effort required to start up these Schemes makes it exceedingly difficult to restart them once they have been stopped. Because of the amount of energy required to start up these Schemes I suggest that it is important not to set up a Pilot Scheme because evaluations have already been done on this way of working, the implications of this type of change are massive and it is much easier to set up Continuity of Carer Schemes throughout the whole area as was done in Riverside Health Authority. The difficult part is setting up, and having gone through that difficult period it is very difficult to engender enough enthusiasm to go through all that again. Pilot Schemes, which invariably consist of a small group of very committed individuals who are often resented because they show up the mediocre care most women are receiving, are always exceedingly vulnerable and one must be aware of this problem and realise how difficult it is to set up such arrangements again.

6

Community-based teams

The woman as the focus of care

The word 'Team' in maternity care has been bandied about and abused so that it has almost become a nonsense word. In 1988 the Association of Radical Midwives, in a letter dated 15 May 1988 sent to all CHCs, RCM Branches, AIMS, NCT, Midwifery Schools and selected MPs, defined more clearly the whole purpose behind continuity of care and Team Schemes:

> We support any scheme in which a woman has the opportunity of getting to know a small number of midwives who will provide her care throughout pregnancy, labour and the postnatal period.

In 'Towards a Healthy Nation' the Royal College of Midwives says:

> The College would strongly support the philosophy that future maternity services be organised so that women experience a continuity of midwifery care.

and

> Local teams of midwives should be established covering specific geographical areas.

Once the woman herself is taken as the pivot around whom care is provided, the focus of care can be seen and recognised –

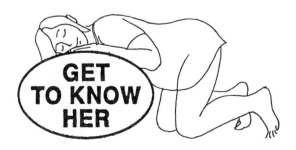

– it is the woman and it is her perception of what her needs are which should be the guide in the provision of care, thus staffing of women becomes the operative modus vivendi – not staffing areas.

In an area when we are not able or not willing to provide 'my midwife', a specific and individual midwife who that woman relates to throughout her pregnancy, labour and puerperium, it is important that we try and base our care on what women have been asking for, so that even if they do not have 'my midwife' they at least have only a small group of midwives they are able to relate to during pregnancy, who are guaranteed to be with them during labour and delivery.

There appear to be different ways of tackling the 'Team' challenge. There are those Teams which are based as much as possible on where the women live – the Community Teams, such as Riverside Community Teams, Oxford Community Teams, Harlow New Town Community Team and Taff/Ely Teams. The other way is to have hospital-based Teams which actually go where the women are – such as the Know Your Midwife Team based at St George's Hospital, Tooting, between 1983 and 1985. There are also hospital-based Teams which would appear to improve the utilisation of midwifery time and skills, but their effect on continuity of care is usually based on chance such as that in the West London Hospital and in Leicester.

Perhaps we should look at a few more examples.

Riverside Midwife Teams

In February 1989 the Riverside Midwife Teams were set up, in the east side of Riverside Health Authority on the north bank of the Thames. The area comprises Westminster, Pimlico, Kensington, Worlds End, Holland Park and Chelsea. In this area of London approximately 1200 women have babies each year, a small number are delivered in private hospitals by private Obstetricians and, of the remainder, the women live in a variety of circumstances.

It is an area of extreme wealth on the one hand and grinding poverty on the other. Large numbers of women live in bed and breakfast hotels or grotty bedsitters, other women live in superb

Team efforts to ease pain of childbirth

MOTHERHOOD

by Ellis Downes

IN the course of a typical pregnancy it is possible for a mother to be seen by more than 30 midwives, nurses, students and medical advisers, many of whom scarcely have time to catch her name, let alone gather any detailed appreciation of her needs.

Next month Riverside health authority in London is expected to give the go-ahead for a radically different approach, known as "continuity of care", which could dramatically improve and humanise the child-bearing experience for all concerned.

"Many women get a lousy deal when they are pregnant", says Caroline Flint, the research midwife, based at the Westminster hospital, who has been largely responsible for devising the new programme. If her proposals are accepted the hours of waiting in crowded antenatal clinics, the delivery by a team of strangers, and the two or three days of postnatal recovery could become things of the past.

Flint says an expectant woman should be cared for, throughout her pregnancy, by the same team of six midwives. During the initial experiment there will be four such teams, each looking after 300 women a year, or roughly six births a week.

When a woman is first pregnant, she will be visited at home by one midwife in the team, whose photograph and biography she will have been sent. The midwife will "book her in" and do routine blood tests. She will then see an obstetrician and have an ultrasound scan. If the pregnancy is normal, as 90% are, all future care will be given either by "her" team or by her own family doctor. Because the specialist obstetricians will see fewer normal pregnancies, they will be able to devote more time to looking after the complicated cases.

By the time the woman is in labour, she will have had about 14 antenatal visits to her own GP, and will know the midwives looking after her. In labour, she will be assessed at home by one of her team who will drive her into hospital. The same midwife will then deliver her baby and take her home, if that is what she wants, no more than six hours later. Any necessary postnatal care will also be provided by the team.

"Why should women have strangers looking after them when they're in labour?" says Flint.

"You don't take strangers on your honeymoon, and labour is far more important." She says research shows that if a woman is assessed in labour at home by someone she knows, she needs less analgesia, is less likely to require caesarean section or forceps delivery, and feels "more in control".

Midwifery morale in Britain is widely recognised to be at an all-time low. Only one in five of the country's midwives is actually working at her chosen job, and there is a 17% national staff shortage. "Midwives are unhappy and they're voting with their feet", says Flint. She has already had many inquiries from midwives about her ideas. They clearly recognise that with continuity of care they would be given more responsibility, learn more and give patients a higher level of support.

Like most positive initiatives, it is not purely altruistic. It will also save money for the health managers, as there will be fewer antenatal hospital admissions, and fewer instrument deliveries, and a sharp reduction in the average hospital stay. As the Riverside health authority is also cutting its maternity beds from 84 to 52, the prospect of discharge six hours after delivery is itself a significant bonus.

Suzanne Truttero, director of midwifery services at the Westminster, believes antenatal care should be decentralised so that low-risk women are given better care.

Final negotiations for the go-ahead of the continuity of care scheme are still taking place, but its widely expected to be approved.

Roger Marwood, consultant obstetrician at the Westminster, says: "We are committed to some form of attempt to change the way we give care." At the moment an obstetrician is responsible for all patient care, but Marwood admitted that "there may well come a time in the future when midwives may be entirely responsible for the care of normal pregnancies".

Flint says: "Being pregnant and giving birth is the best experience a woman can ever have. I want to make it a lot better."

Reproduced, with permission from the author, from Downes, 1988.

and palatial houses with staff and a nanny, other women live in army Barracks. The women are English, Irish, Eastern European, Arabic, Afro-caribbean, Asian, Malaysian, Jewish, American, a fascinating mixture of cultures and creeds.

The women either go to the local GP to report their pregnancy or to the local Health Authority Clinic where the midwives are based. In the area are four teams, each consisting of six midwives or WTEs (whole time equivalents), thus one of the Teams has seven midwives because two of the midwives are job sharing. The midwives are based in local centres where the Health Visitors are also based. Each Midwife Team has responsibility for approximately 250–300 women a year, the women are given a photograph and description of their Team members and during their pregnancy they will meet the six midwives.

The woman has her booking done in her own home, but from then onwards she comes to the Midwives' Clinic for her follow-on antenatal care. She may see an Obstetrician at the hospital once, not at all, twice or on alternate visits depending on her medical needs. The same happens with her GP who she may see once, not at all, or at regular intervals.

All the midwives carry long range message pagers and are able to receive quite long messages from each other and from the women. The women are all given the number of their Team and can bleep them at any time of the day or night.

When a woman goes into labour she bleeps her Team and the midwife on call responds. Most women are assessed at home in early labour and then transferred into the West London Hospital for delivery unless they are booked for a home birth when they stay at home. The midwife she knows stays with her throughout her labour but if the time becomes very prolonged the midwife from the Team who takes over the woman's care is also known to her, so she is never attended by strangers.

Once the woman has delivered she either goes home, or she transfers to the Postnatal Ward where she will be visited daily by the Midwife Team. This care continues once she has gone home.

Thus in this area of London all women, whatever their 'risk' status, receive care from midwives they are able to get to know. The Scheme has been evaluated with reference to the amount of intervention women are experiencing compared to before the Scheme started, the levels of staff satisfaction when working in the Teams compared with hospital staff both before the Teams started and at the hospital now, costs are being evaluated, it cost in the region of £64 000 to set up the Teams but it enabled a Maternity Unit (at the Westminster Hospital) to be closed, so saving several million pounds, and the cost of the antenatal care has been calculated by the Finance Department within the Health Authority to be £140 cheaper per woman compared with both GP shared care and Hospital antenatal care. At the time of writing it is very hard to work out costings within the NHS as they are in the process of being calculated but an attempt, which is believed to be as accurate as possible, has been described on pp. 55 and 58.

The midwives in the Riverside Scheme are either on call during the day from 9 a.m. to 6 p.m., when they work with their colleagues – handing over any work if they are called to a labouring woman. At night they do a run of on calls (usually five in a row) when they are on call from 6 p.m. until 9 a.m., during the day they rest at home if they were called the preceding night but if they weren't they come in to do a Booking or to help at an Antenatal Clinic. The midwives calculate the length of time they are called for and claim the appropriate rate if they are called during the night, during a Bank Holiday, etc. The hours the midwives work are flexible in that they keep a record of how many hours they work and are paid back if they work too many (over 150 hours every 4 weeks).

The Teams contain six midwives – these midwives provide all antenatal and postnatal care for the women who live in their area, and all the women are looked after in labour and delivered by a midwife they know. The only women who don't receive this care are those whose GPs have deflected them to another hospital on the south side of the Thames (there are a group of GPs who have tried to sabotage this system) or if they are booked with a private Obstetrician for delivery in a Private Obstetric Unit.

The scheme was set up in order to improve maternity care in that area and it has been running successfully for over 3½ years. The brief for setting up the Teams was:

1. To increase continuity of care for women.
2. To increase midwives' job satisfaction.

The Teams have achieved both of these aims.

Taff Ely/Rhondda Teams

In the Rhondda Valley in South Wales on 1 September 1987, inspired by the then Director of Midwifery Services Jean Cushing, another scheme called the 'Know Your Midwife' Scheme was set up in the valleys around Cardiff. Between 250 and 300 women a year were to receive antenatal, delivery and postnatal care from a Team of six midwives they had been able to get to know during their pregnancy.

In this Scheme, when a woman books, she is booked with one of the Team midwives and is given a photograph and details of all six of the midwives in her Team. Some of the comments from the midwives with their photos are: "I am from Hampshire but have moved to the Rhondda to take part in the 'Know Your Midwife' Scheme and now look forward to meeting you all."; "I have moved to the Rhondda from Nottingham especially to take part in the 'Know Your Midwife' Scheme. My young children have settled down really well in the Rhondda."; "I am Rhondda born and bred and have been practising Midwifery for four years."

The women in the scheme had been used to using the local Unit, Llwynypia Hospital, for delivery but over the years the Unit had done less and less deliveries, resulting in only 100 per year being performed prior to the advent of the KYM Scheme. The Antenatal Clinic in the small Unit has been updated so that women are seen in privacy and there are ultrasound facilities on site. Women were being seen by Consultants from East Glamorgan Hospital in the Antenatal Clinic in Llwynypia Hospital, then they were also seeing their GPs and they were delivering in East Glamorgan Hospital, meeting totally strange midwives when they went into the hospital in labour. The KYM Scheme was set up in order to enable the women to get to know their Team of six midwives antenatally. When they go into labour they telephone their midwives who usually visit them at home to assess the progress of the labour.

The Teams have developed since their inception – there are now seven midwives on each Team – 6½ WTEs.

Once labour is established, midwife, labouring mother, husband and any other companions go to East Glamorgan Hospital for the delivery (unless the woman is booked for a home delivery – the numbers of which are increasing). The woman comes home when she decides to and is again looked after by her midwives. If her delivery is complicated all the midwives can assist at an instrumented delivery or scrub for a caesarean section, or scrub up to take the baby, so they are able to provide the mother's care throughout her labour, whatever the outcome.

The initial pilot scheme was so successful that by 1992 five teams were working in Taff Ely/Rhondda. They care for between 220 and 280 women a year for each Team. Each Team has seven midwives (6.5 WTEs).

The Teams of midwives deliver care to the women in their homes, in the GP's surgery, in Midwives' Clinics, Hospital Antenatal Clinics, Hospital Wards, Delivery Suite, Theatre, wherever the woman happens to be – they are woman based rather than ward based.

In November 1989 the results of an evaluation of the first year of the first Rhondda Team's work was presented to the Health Authority. The results were summarised thus:

1. Communication improved with KYM.
2. Expectation of pain in labour closer to reality.
3. Assessment of the success of self-help techniques more optimistic and closer to that of the patient.
4. KYM women felt that a midwife was available whenever they needed her.
5. The women are in the hospital for a shorter time preceding delivery.
6. KYM midwives less likely to perform an episiotomy.
7. Less fetal distress, but number of cases not statistically significant.
8. APGAR scores higher.
9. Percentage of mothers delivered by Team midwives was much greater than that achieved by other KYM schemes.
10. Increased satisfaction by midwives.
11. Did not diminish the need for a partner or friend at delivery.
12. Women were less likely to make adverse comments regarding the staff or the environment.
13. Higher uptake of immunisation.

(Jean Cushing, Director of Midwifery, Clinical Practice and Research, 6 November 1989, personal communication.)

Further evaluation has taken place since Jean Keats has taken over as Director of Midwifery Services, undertaken by the University of Wales College of Medicine, and showed:

- KYM women had fewer admissions to hospital in the antenatal period than women in the control group.
- KYM women had a lower episiotomy rate than women in the control group.
- KYM women showed higher attendance at antenatal classes.
- KYM women made more positive comments and fewer adverse comments on care during labour and delivery.
- KYM women were more likely to accept all infant immunisations at 6 weeks than were the controls.

One of the fascinating aspects of different Teams is that they all develop differently. One of the Taff Ely/Rhondda Teams is the Taff/Ely Domino Team which works differently from the other Teams in that it offers delivery only to low-risk women and there are only four midwives in that Team, they have now joined forces with two hospital-based midwives – one on night duty and one on day duty. This means that when one of these midwives is on duty the Community Midwife does not have to come in with their woman, she is looked after by the midwife based in the hospital. The women are invited to coffee mornings, antenatal classes and aquanatal classes in order to get to know the six midwives, whose caseload is 300 women a year (but the high-risk women in the 300 are only receiving antenatal and mainly postnatal care from the midwives).

Although the Taff/Ely Domino Team has not been in operation for very long some interesting data has already been collected:

- Consumer satisfaction rates are increased.
- There is a higher uptake of preparation classes.
- Ninety-one per cent of mothers who started by breastfeeding have continued up to and beyond the eighth week.

(Results from Jean Keats, Manager Maternal and Child Health from a speech given at the Royal College of Midwives Professional Day Conference Friday 24 July 1992.)

The significance of Wales as being in the forefront of excellent maternity care should not be ignored. In 1988 the Secretary of State for Wales set up the Welsh Health Planning

Forum as an advisory subgroup of the Executive Committee of the Health Policy Board of the NHS. In August 1991 it reported and set out its Protocol for Investment in Health Gain in Maternal and Child Health, this document is one of several covering different aspects of health care – the objective being to develop 'health gains', i.e. to improve the health of the population by specific interventions.

Para 7   As a consequence of the past drive for health gain with its emphasis on the safety of mother and child, there has been a reduction in the options available to mothers and an increase in medical involvement and interventions. There is now a view, shared by the NHS, that mothers should be given more **choice** and more **control** over the process, and that the *people centred focus* should be strengthened.

Para 100   *Continuity of care* with known and trusted carers available to the mother before, during and after the birth, has been shown to increase satisfaction with the service offered and also improves understanding and confidence among mothers. A recent overview of studies focusing on Childbirth recommended that forms of care which do not provide continuity of care should be abandoned.

Para 203   If a woman is to give birth successfully she has to have confidence in herself and in those who will be attending at the birth. Continuity of care has been shown to promote this. Some will want a partnership with the professional staff involved, others may not.

Para 290   A positive experience of childbirth is important in determining the mother's attitude to her child and her family. This goes far beyond simple satisfaction with the services offered, and requires the service to be truly people centred.

Para 306   Continuity of carer enables women to build up relationships of trust, and feel able to ask questions, understand what is happening and participate in decisions concerning their care. There are a number of ways in which this can be achieved, including the DOMINO scheme, the Know Your Midwife approach, care by a GP maternity unit, and continuous care of high risk women by consultant obstetricians. Although supported by WHO and research in the United Kingdom, it is not the norm, and needs to be pursued.

MAUREEN FREELY

Assembly-line health service economies that fail to deliver

ONE OF the arguments against last month's Benetton new-born baby-cum-umbilical cord ad was that it was a commercialisation of what was meant to be a private event. Where did they get that idea?

When I gave birth to my first child in a London teaching hospital, I had two dozen student midwives in attendance. When I gave birth to my second, I had so many doctors and nurses arguing over my bed that I thought I had died and woken up on the set of a soap opera. I was a prop, there to generate worrying foetal heartbeat graphs and to add to the suspense by contriving to get myself stuck in the lift on the way to the operating theatre. My husband did his best to try and remind the people that I could hear everything they were saying, but the odds were against us, especially when it emerged that the anaesthetist on duty was out playing golf without his bleeper. Although our daughter was (eventually) born healthy, neither of us has ever fully recovered from the birth.

The classic way of explaining the distress felt by women after a birth that deviates from the ideal is that she is ashamed of not having performed well, but I would say that my shame after an emergency Caesarean came from my sense that I had lost control. I had gone into hospital to give birth to a child. Instead I had that child taken away from me. I was the only person who seemed to realise what had happened. Everyone else told me how happy I ought to be that they had "managed to get her out in time". I felt the same kind of dislocation years later in hospital after a miscarriage. Though the doctors and nurses went out of their way to make the service personal by explaining exactly what my operation would entail, they didn't question the dreadful hospital policy of putting the miscarriages in the same ward as the terminations, nor the horrible name of the procedure to which I was to be subjected (Evacuation of the Products of Conception). These were the organisational flaws that caused us the most distress and left the biggest scars.

It doesn't have to be that way, as I discovered to my surprise when I went into hospital to have my new baby girl earlier this month. This time I was in the care of a midwife I had first met seven months ago, and who I had already come to trust as a friend. She belongs to a six-woman team (the second to have been set up by the NHS in the Oxford area) which establishes contact with its patients from the day they make their first antenatal visit to the GP. The team is based at the hospital and has someone on call 24 hours a day. It also does weekly antenatal clinics in conjunction with the family doctors who refer patients to the team. It runs its own birth classes, visits the home towards the end of the last trimester, undertakes to supervise early labour in the home if appropriate, sees deliveries through, whether they are at home or in hospital, and continues to look after both mother and child during the 10 days following the birth.

They will continue these daily home visits for as long as there are problems. If they left the timing of the final discharge to me, it would never happen. I can see us sitting over coffee, two or three years from now discussing playgroups and nutrition with the same interest that we now discuss pelvic tilts and the strange reactions people can have to the name Helen. Of course, this is just the type of fantasy that drives critics of team midwifery — and there are lots of them in our local health authority — round the bend.

The NHS is not in the business of providing cosy chats, they say. What they don't seem to realise is that what seems like a cosy chat to me is conversation in the line of duty for the midwife. I am sure, for example, that my midwife Aileen's idea of a relaxing day is not sitting in a windowless delivery room listening to me groan along to the World Saxophone Quartet. But, because people are allowed to bring in the music of their choice, she pretended to enjoy it as much as my boyfriend and I did. If the conversation she engaged us in between contractions was at times pleasant enough for us to forget where we were and why, then this too was good medical practice because we were then calm enough to hear her instructions and trusted her enough to follow them closely. If it turned out to be a text-book birth, it was partly simple good luck but it was also thanks to careful management. I am sure that if she had been present at the other two births they would have been shorter, with fewer complications, and therefore less traumatic.

That is all very well, say the critics but the service is an unnecessary expense. What I say in response is that it is expensive only because it is a pilot programme. If they reorganised all their midwives into teams they would be able to make it financially viable. The number of hours I spent in care to have my first two children was far greater than this time – partly because I suffered complications at times when I was unobserved because midwives were changing shifts, or when underqualified nurses were standing in for missing doctors.

It's also obvious that a service which provides continuity of care instead of assembly-line medicine will be able to identify problems earlier and so cut down on expensive interventions. A mother who has been well supported before birth and who has not had to hand her body over to strangers during labour, is more likely to be able to stand on her own feet afterwards and less likely to become an NHS burden in the years that follow. Unfortunately, the engineers of the new, improved health service don't seem to have been able to assign a numerical value to quality care – and this despite paying lip service to preventive medicine. And so it doesn't show up on their balance sheets, which they continue to draw up according to business concepts so narrow and old-fashioned that even an Italian clothing company would find them laughable. If Benetton had really wanted to promote the commercialised birth, they ought to have run a poster of the white paper.

Oxford

In Oxford, Community Midwives in the centre of the city have been providing women with continuity of carer for many years. In 1966, 40% of women were delivered at home by Oxford's Community Midwives (personal communication with Chloe Fisher, Senior Midwife) – this figure was slightly higher, but more or less in line, with the rest of the country. The Cranbrook report of 1957 had proposed a 70% hospital delivery rate.

The Cranbrook Report had also suggested integration of Hospital, Community and GP services – and in Oxford, in order to comply with this suggestion, in August 1966 a GP Unit was set up within the main hospital and the 40% of women who up to that time had had home deliveries were encouraged to be delivered there by the Community Midwives in the GP Unit.

The GP Unit was for very low-risk women, it was presumed that the other 60% of women would be looked after in the Consultant Unit with most of them having shared care with the GP and the Community Midwife attached to his practice. When these women go into labour they go to the Hospital where they are likely to meet midwives they do not know and be looked after by them throughout their labour.

Today this system still operates – in central Oxford there are about 2000 women who give birth each year, in 1989 about 1000 of those women were booked by the Community Midwives for delivery. The Community Midwives work in pairs, each pair works in a Team of six, there are three such Groups of midwives. About 25% of women are transferred out of Community Midwife care over to Consultant Unit care.

Those women delivered by their primary Community Midwife or her partner made up 60% of the remaining women. Most of the remaining 40% were delivered by someone else in the Group of Community Midwives who they may or may not have met before.

The midwives are on call for 'their' women throughout the day while they are working. At night they do a 1 in 3–4 rota when they are on call for the women from the whole Group of six midwives.

In Chapter 3 I describe a study by Klein *et al.* (1983a,b) which showed the benefits of such care for women. The study shows the differences that occur when women are assessed at home during early labour by midwives. The difference this home assessment makes has enormous benefits for women and their babies.

Kidlington Midwifery Team, Oxford

A scheme to provide women with greater continuity of care was organised in this part of Oxfordshire by Lesley Page (now Professor Lesley Page), then the Director of Midwifery Services at the John Radcliffe Hospital. In February 1989 a Team of five full-time midwives and one 0.8 part-time midwife began to work in the Kidlington area of Oxford. The midwives were based in the John Radcliffe Hospital in Oxford and they were initially attached to the GPs working in the two local Health Centres in Kidlington; they are now also attached to a GP practice in Islip, and they look after all the women of Kidlington and Islip during their pregnancies, go to the woman's house when she calls when she is in labour, and when the time is ready they go together to the John Radcliffe Hospital in Oxford for delivery in the Delivery Unit. The Team has now grown to five full-time midwives, two midwives who are job sharing, and one part-time midwife.

Unless they want to go home immediately after delivery the women are transferred to the Postnatal Ward at the John Radcliffe Hospital. They are visited daily by the midwife from their Team. Once the women go home from the hospital, either within a few hours of delivery or a few days following delivery, their Team of midwives will carry out their postnatal care at home – midwives they know and feel towards as friends.

The pregnant women are encouraged to get to know all six midwives in the Team, they know that they may have any one of those midwives to care for them during labour. The midwives are on call for 24 hours, and they come in to work from the Unit during the day when they are on call, and if they are called to a woman in labour they transfer the work they were going to do to one of their colleagues.

Harlow

Pauline Wells, Assistant Director in the Directorate of Obstetrics and Gynaecology in Harlow, Essex reports on the scheme set up in Harlow New Town which is operating from a GP Health Centre with seven midwives based in the Centre. The midwifery practice is called the Mayer Practice in memory of a former Harlow midwife, Sister Diane Mayer. The seven midwives carry bleepers, the women are able to get to know the seven midwives and are assured that one of them will be delivering their baby when they go into labour. Because of the bleepers the women have access at all times to a midwife who they know. Following delivery many of the women are only in hospital for 6 hours and they are looked after by the same Team of midwives when they come home.

The Team had 95 births in their first 3 months, which is an average of one birth a day. The women are appreciating the care they are receiving and the midwives are being encouraged to hold weekly meetings in order to help them to develop as a Team and to smooth out any problems they might have. It is seen as a pilot scheme for the whole of Essex and Herts in which there are 3000 deliveries every year, the aim being to bring this type of care to all pregnant women in the whole Health Authority.

The plan is that from September 1992 all the midwives will be community based and that this scheme will be available to all the women in the Health Authority.

Scunthorpe

On 30 July 1990 the Winterton Practice of four midwives and one bank midwife set up a continuity of carer scheme in Winterton in Lincolnshire. The team of midwives are based in a GP's surgery and they deliver between 140 and 200 women a year. The Scheme has been enormously popular with women, who are able to get to know the four midwives during their pregnancies either through their antenatal checks, their antenatal classes or a monthly 'pop-in' session when all the midwives are available.

Many of the benefits already described as ensuing from continuity of carer have happened with this team. First, Category X patients have been greatly reduced, i.e. when a woman goes into labour she bleeps the midwife on call who then goes to the woman's house to assess her in labour. From August 1990 to January 1991 164 mothers were assessed at home, and of these 73 required admission while 91 remained at home having been checked by the midwife, thus a potential saving of 91 intranatal inpatient days was saved.

The number of antenatal admissions between August 1990 and January 1991 was only four from the women looked after by the Team, compared with 444 from other areas served by Scunthorpe General Hospital. No women looked after by the midwives in the Scheme were readmitted with postnatal complications and no babies needed special care nursing. The average postnatal stay for the women being looked after in the Team was 2.5 days compared with 3.5 days for other mothers. Amazingly 80.8% of mothers within the scheme breastfed compared with 30% of other women being looked after in the Maternity Unit at Scunthorpe General Hospital.

There was an increase in travelling costs, mileage costs approximately doubled from the days when Community Midwives did mainly postnatal care, but it was expected that the cost saving in antenatal beds and admissions and the reduced postnatal stay would have counterbalanced the increased cost of mileage. One interesting comment in the evaluation is that having set up a Team of midwives it had inadvertently resulted in two types of midwife within the Labour Ward, one who was allowed to practise autonomously, with medical intervention given only when requested by the midwives. For the remaining mothers and babies in the hospital accountability appeared to be with the medical staff. Thus the midwives in the Winterton Team were seen as being responsible enough by the medical staff to be able to organise their own work and to take full responsibility for the care of labouring mothers, which was not the case with the other Labour Ward Midwives.

Since the implementation of the first Midwifery Team a further four Teams were set up and in January 1993, the intention is that this will be increased to ten Teams to cover the whole Health District.

In the examples given of duty rotas, if I know where the rotas have come from I acknowledge the source, if I think that I devised them myself obviously I leave that blank. If there is one here that I think that I have devised and you think that you devised it, please write to me c/o the publisher and with the next reprint we will acknowledge your contribution. Our obsession as a profession with pieces of squared paper fascinates me and I have collected dozens over the years and I don't always know where they originally came from.

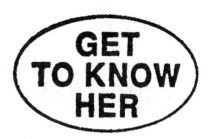

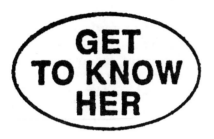

7

Duty rotas

Every Team develops its own unique way of working, every pair of midwives in partnership develops its own modus vivendi. The following examples of rotas are to give you ideas and to help you to decide what sort of way you could work and for others to decide whether anyone else could work with you in the same sort of set-up. I hope they will be of some help, some have been used successfully, some are ideas and examples culled over the years from my travels around the world to Birth Centres in Australia, Japan and the United States, and from talking with midwives in State Health and Independent Practices both here and abroad.

There would appear to be some guiding principles when making up a duty rota. First that for whatever number of midwives there are in a Team or Group the rota must be done for one less person than there is in actuality. For instance, if there are four midwives in a Group Practice the rota must be done for three, likewise if there is a Team of six the rota must be set out for five, this is because at any time there will be one person on holiday, away on a course or other activity.

It would seem only sensible that the rota should be on-going, a rhythm that repeats itself over and over again. This means that people can look at the rota and know what they will be doing on Saturday in 8 weeks' time, and if that duty is not convenient they can swap with a colleague in good time. One of the most constant complaints of midwives when I visit them in different parts of the United Kingdom is that they don't know what their off duties are far enough in advance and that often they find it impossible to organise their social life except at the last minute – this is very unsatisfactory, it stops midwives developing outside interests in their spare time, it impedes on-going education in free time, it stops the midwives from joining regular clubs and courses and is extremely restricting.

There is of course the counter argument, that midwives like to know their off duty in advance because they like request the evenings off that they want and the days off, so each week the off duty must be re-invented and worked at from scratch. I would suggest that this compliance to the present system is to do with women making the best of the situation they find themselves in, it is an example of how they manage to cope with an unacceptable practice and then begin to perceive as the best, or only, alternative.

Once midwives know that their off duty is going to be for weeks and weeks in advance life opens up considerably. We only have to look at other groups who have to provide 24-hour cover to see that it can be done efficiently. Firemen know their duty rosters for 12 months in advance, telephonists in an international news agency know their duty rosters for 12 weeks in advance, bus drivers and conductors have 13-week rosters as do motormen and guards on the railways and London Transport underground. It seems to be only nurses and midwives who spend hours every week working out next week's off duty, with a list of 'requests' in one hand and a large squared sheet in the other. Did you really train for three or four and a half years to do this?

The other principle is that if an off-duty rota is for seven midwives then it will repeat itself every 7 weeks, if for six – then every 6 weeks.

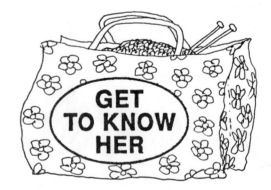

Team of Six

	M	Tu	W	Th	F	S	S	M	Tu	W	Th	F	S	S	M	Tu	W	Th	F	S	S
	D	oc	L	E	oc	E	D	L	E	D	E	E	D	oc	E	E	L	oc	D	E	E
	D	E	oc	L	E	E	D	E	oc	E	E	D	D	D	E	E	L	E	D	oc	E
	E	E	E	L	L	oc	E	D	D	E	L	E	D	D	oc	L	E	E	E	D	D
	E	D	E	oc	D	E	oc	L	L	E	E	oc	E	E	D	E	oc	L	L	D	E
	oc	L	D	E	oc	D	E	E	E	E	L	E	oc	E	L	D	oc	L	D	D	oc
				COVER FOR ANNUAL LEAVE, OVERTIME, REFRESHER COURSES ETC.							PROPOSED										

	M	Tu	W	Th	F	S	S	M	Tu	W	Th	F	S	S	M	Tu	W	Th	F	S	S
	E	E	D	L	L	D	E	oc	E	E	L	E	D	D	E	D	L	oc	E	D	D
	E	oc	E	L	E	D	E	E	E	L	E	D	D	D	D	E	E	E	oc	D	D
	L	L	D	E	E	D	L	E	E	oc	L	D	oc	E	L	L	E	E	D	oc	E
	E	E	E	L	E	E	oc	D	D	D	oc	D	E	D	oc	oc	E	L	L	E	oc
	E	D	L	oc	E	D	D	L	L	oc	E	D	E	E	oc	E	E	L	E	D	D
	oc				SHIFT PATTERN 1				REFRESHER COURSES						ETC.						

PROPOSED SHIFT PATTERN 1

With this off duty there is only one midwife on call but she can call on one of her colleagues by mutual agreement if she needs her.

E = EARLY SHIFT   09.00–17.00. Early shift midwives do all the postnatal care of women on the scheme, plus Booking visits (6–7 a week)

L = LATE SHIFT   13.00–21.00. All antenatal care is done by the late shift midwife either in a Clinic or in a woman's home. Booking visits in the home are divided up between late and early shift midwives

OC = ON CALL   On call is from midnight until midnight the following day. The midwife needs to be available for anyone in labour or anyone with a problem

D = DAY OFF

THE 6th MIDWIFE   Has no set shift pattern, but is available to cover absences due to annual leave, refresher courses, overtime owing to the other midwives and sick leave

Team of Six

	M	Tu	W	Th	F	S	S	M	Tu	W	Th	F	S	S	M	Tu	W	Th	F	S	S	M	Tu	W	Th	F	S	S	M	Tu	W	Th	F	S	S	M	Tu	W	Th	F	S	S
	OC	L	D	L	E	E	OC	E	D	L	E	E	D	OC	D	L	OC	E	E	D	D	OC	L	D	E	E	D	OC	L	E	OC	E	E	D	D	L	D	D	L	E	E	OC
	E	E	D	E	E	D	D	L	E	D	E	E	OC	D	L	OC	E	E	D	D	E	D	E	L	E	E	OC	D	OC	L	E	E	D	D	L	OC	E	E	D	L	L	E
	E	D	L	E	E	D	D	D	D	D	L	D	E	D	OC	E	E	D	L	OC	D	D	L	OC	E	D	E	D	E	E	L	D	L	E	E	D	L	E	E	D	D	D
	D	L	E	D	E	D	D	E	L	E	E	D	D	E	E	D	L	D	D	E	L	L	E	E	D	L	D	D	E	E	D	L	OC	L	E	E	D	D	OC	E	E	D
	L	OC	E	L	OC	E	E	E	OC	E	OC	L	L	E	E	E	D	L	OC	E	OC	E	D	D	L	OC	L	D	E	D	E	OC	L	OC	OC	D	OC	L	E	OC	OC	OC

COVER FOR HOLIDAYS, REFRESHER COURSES, OVERTIME, SICK LEAVE ETC.

PROPOSED SHIFT PATTERN 2

PROPOSED SHIFT PATTERN 2

With this off duty there is only one midwife on call but she can call on one of her colleagues by mutual agreement if she need her.

E = EARLY SHIFT   09.00–17.00. Early shift midwives do all the postnatal care of women on the scheme, plus Booking visits (6–7 a week)

L = LATE SHIFT   13.00–21.00. All antenatal care is done by the late shift midwife either in a Clinic or in a woman's home. Booking visits in the home are divided up between late and early shift midwives

OC = ON CALL   On call is from 09.00 until 09.00 the following day. The midwife needs to be available for anyone in labour or anyone with a problem

D = DAY OFF

THE 6th MIDWIFE   Has no set shift pattern, but is available to cover absences due to annual leave, refresher courses, overtime owing to the other midwives and sick leave

Team of Six

	M	Tu	W	Th	F	S	S	M	Tu	W	Th	F	S	S	M	Tu	W	Th	F	S	S	M	Tu	W	Th	F	S	S
	OC	L	E	OC	L	OC	E	D	L	E	OC	L	OC	E	D	L	E	OC	L	OC	E	D	L	E	OC	L	OC	E
	L	E	L	D	E	E	OC	L	OC	E	E	D	E	D	L	OC	E	E	D	E	D	L	OC	E	E	D	D	D
	E	L	E	L	D	OC	D	OC	L	D	D	L	D	D	OC	L	D	D	L	D	D	OC	OC	L	D	L	D	D
	E	E	L	E	E	D	D	E	E	E	E	OC	E	E	D	E	E	OC	E	E	D	D	E	E	E	E	OC	D
	D	D	OC	E	E	D	D	L	E	D	L	E	OC	E	E	D	L	E	OC	E	E	D	D	E	L	D	OC	E
	L	E	D	E	OC	D	E	E	D	OC	E	E	D	OC	L	E	D	OC	E	E	D	L	E	D	D	E	E	OC

No long spans

COVER FOR ANNUAL LEAVE, REFRESHER COURSES, OVERTIME, SICK LEAVE ETC.

PROPOSED SHIFT PATTERN 3

PROPOSED SHIFT PATTERN 3

With this off duty there is only one midwife on call but she can call on one of her colleagues by mutual agreement if she needs her. This off duty has been designed so that there are no long spans in it.

E = EARLY SHIFT   09.00–17.00. Early shift midwives do all the postnatal care of women on the scheme, plus Booking visits (6–7 a week)

L = LATE SHIFT   13.00–21.00. All antenatal care is done by the late shift midwife either in a Clinic or in a woman's home. Booking visits in the home are divided up between late and early shift midwives

OC = ON CALL   On call is from 09.00 until 09.00 the following day. The midwife needs to be available for anyone in labour or anyone with a problem

D = DAY OFF

THE 6th MIDWIFE   Has no set shift pattern, but is available to cover absences due to annual leave, refresher courses, overtime owing to the other midwives and sick leave

Team of Six

S	M	Tu	W	Th	F	S	S	M	Tu	W	Th	F	S	S	M	Tu	W	Th	F	S	S	M	Tu	W	Th	F	S	S	M	Tu	W	Th	F	S
D	2	C/H	C/H	1	2	1	C/H	1	D	C/H	2	1	1	C/H	1	2	C/H	D	1	D	D	1	2	C/H	C/H	1	2	1	C/H	C/H	1	C/H	2	D
D	1	2	1	2	C/H	1	C/H	D	C/H	D	D	1	D	D	1	2	D	2	1	D	D	2	D	D	D	1	D	D	2	D	1	C/H	1	D
D	D	1	C/H	2	C/H	C/H	C/H	D	C/H	C/H	C/H	C/H	1	C/H	D	C/H	C/H	C/H	1	1	D	D	C/H	C/H	C/H	C/H	1	C/H	C/H	C/H	C/H	C/H	C/H	C/H
D	D	D	C/H	D	1	C/H	D	D	1	D	2	2	2	D	D	1	D	2	2	1	D	1	2	D	C/H	2	D	D	D	2	1	1	2	C/H
1	C/H	C/H	C/H	C/H	D	2	1	D	D	1	1	1	1	C/H	2	1	C/H	1	C/H	D	2	2	1	D	2	1	D	2	1	1	D	2	1	1
C/H	C/H	C/H	1	C/H	C/H	D	C/H	C/H	1	1	2	2	1	2	C/H	1	2	2	C/H	D	1	C/H	1	2	1	C/H	D	C/H	C/H	1	2	D	2	1

COVER FOR ANNUAL LEAVE, REFRESHER COURSES, OVERTIME, SICK LEAVE ETC.

PROPOSED SHIFT PATTERN 4

3 weekends every 5 weeks

PROPOSED SHIFT PATTERN 4

With this off duty there are two midwives on call and each midwife has three weekends off every 5 weeks.

C/H = COMMUNITY + HOSPITAL   Either 09.00–17.00 or 13.00–21.00 as appropriate. These midwives do all the postnatal care of women on the scheme, both in hospital and the community. They are also responsible for Antenatal Consultations of women in the scheme

1 = FIRST ON CALL
2 = SECOND ON CALL

On call is from 09.00 until 09.00 the following day. The midwife needs to be available for anyone in labour or anyone with a problem. The Second On Call midwife does a Booking visit every day and two on one day a week – she also carries out Antenatal Consultations as necessary

D = DAY OFF

THE 6th MIDWIFE   Has no set shift pattern, but is available to cover absences due to annual leave, refresher courses, overtime owing to the other midwives and sick leave

The original Know Your Midwife Rota (Team of Four)
(Source: *Nursing Times* 30 January 1985)

THE TEAM FROM TOOTING

Mon	Tues	Wed	Thur	Fri	Sat	Sun	Mon	Tues	Wed	Thur	Fri	Sat	Sun	Mon
DO	DO	OC	E	OC	1/2	OC	E	OC	E	DO	DO	OC	1/2	OC
E	OC	E	DO	DO	OC	1/2	OC	E	1-9	OC	E	DO	DO	DO
OC	E	1-9	OC	E	DO	DO	DO	OC	OC	E	OC	1/2	OC	E
*	*	*	*	*	*	*	*	*	*	*	*	*	*	*

Tue	Wed	Thur	Fri	Sat	Sun
E	1-9	OC	E	DO	DO
DO	OC	E	OC	1/2	OC
OC	E	DO	DO	OC	1/2
*	*	*	*	*	*

The rota repeats itself every three weeks –
the fourth midwife (*) fills in for holidays and
time owed

and how it worked in practice

Know Your Midwife Team

MONTH BEGINNING: MAY 6th 1984   HOSPITAL:

NAME AND INITIAL (Block Caps)	GRADE/YEAR	DATE	6	7	8	9	10	11	12	13	14	15	16	17	18	19	20	21	22	23	24	25	26	27	28	29	30	31	1
		HRS	S	M	Tu	W	Th	F	S	S	M	Tu	W	Th	F	S	S	M	Tu	W	Th	F	S	S	M	Tu	W	Th	F
Caroline FLINT	SR			E									✗																	
Penny CHURCH	SM		1/2D	oc	E	1-9	oc	E	DO	DO	D	D	D	E	oc	1/2D	oc	E	oc	E	oc	E	1/2D	oc	oc	E	1-9	oc	E
Claire NEIL	SM		D	D	D	oc	E	D	1/2D	oc	E	D	oc	E	D	AL	AL	AL	AL	AL	AL	AL	D	D	D	D	oc	E	D
Wendy PEARCE	SM		oc	BH	D	oc	D	D	oc	oc	oc	E	1-9	oc	E	D	D	D	D	oc	E	oc	AL	AL	AL	AL	AL	AL	D

JUNE

Team of Six: community based

S	M	T	W	T	F	S	S	M	T	W	T	F	S	S	M	T	W	T	F	S	S	M	T	W	T	F	S	S	M	T	W	T	F	S	S	M	T	W	T	F	S
1	2	E	E	E	E	T		E₂ 1	L	E	1	E	E		E₂ 1	E	L	E	E	2		1	E	E	E	2	E	1	E₂	E	2	E	E	E	1		2	E	1		E	E₂
E₂	1	1	E	E	1	E₂ 1	1	E	2	E		E	1	E₂ 1	L	1	E	2	E	E₂ 1	2	L	1	2	E	L	1	E₂	L	E	2	E	L	2	E₂ 1	E	E	2	1	2	1
	2	1	E	E	E	E₂ 1	E	2	E	2	E	E	2	E₂ 1	E	E	1	E	2	1	E	E	E	1	E	E	L	E	L	2	E	E	E	L	E₂ 1	E	L	2	E	E	1
E₂	1	L	1	2	2	1	2	1	2		1	1	E₂ 1	E 1	E 2	E 1	E 1	E 1	E 2	E 1	E₂ 1	E 2	E 1	E 2	L	E 2	E 1	E 1	E 2	E 1	E 2	E E	E 1	E E	E 1	L 1	E L	E 2	E E	E 1	E 1

COVER FOR AL, OVERTIME, SICKNESS + REFRESHER COURSES

E = 9 a.m.–5 p.m. Antenatal and postnatal care in community and hospital

L = 1 p.m.– 9 p.m. Antenatal and postnatal care in community and hospital

$\left.\begin{array}{c} 1 \\ 2 \end{array}\right\}$ = First and Second On Call from 9 a.m. to 9 a.m. On Call for labouring women and any problems or queries

E₂ = 9 a.m. until necessary plus Second On Call

■ = Day off

Acknowledgements to Holland Street Team.

Team of Six: community based

Day					
M	L	L	E	1	2
Tu	E	E	1	2	E
W		2	E	1	
Th		E	1	2	
F	1	E	E	2	E
S	E₂	1			
S	1	E₂			
M	2	1	E	L	L
Tu	E	2	E	1	E
W	E	1	2		
Th	2	E		1	
F	E	E	1	E	2
S	1	E₂			
S	E₂	1			
M	L	1	2	E	L
Tu	E	2	E	1	E
W	E	1	2		
Th	1	2	E		
F	E	2	E	E	1
S	1	E₂			
S	E₂	1			
M	E	L	L	1	2
Tu	1	E	E	2	E
W	2	E	1		
Th	E	1	2		
F	E	E	1	2	E
S	1	E₂			
S	E₂	1			
M	1	E	2	L	L
Tu	2	1	E	E	E
W	E	2	1		
Th	1	E	2		
F	2	E	E	E	1
S	1	E₂			

COVER FOR AL, STUDY LEAVE ETC.

E = 9 a.m.–5 p.m. Antenatal and postnatal care in community and hospital

L = 1 p.m.–9 p.m. Antenatal and postnatal care in community and hospital

1⎫
2⎭ = On Call – First and Second from 9 a.m. to 9 a.m. On Call for labouring women and any problems or queries

E₂ = 9 a.m. until necessary plus Second On Call

■ = Day off

Acknowledgements to Bessborough Street Team.

Team of Six: community based

Day	1	2	3	4	5	6
M	N		D		I	C
Tu	*	N	D	D	L	C
W	*	N	D	D	AL	C
Th	N		D	■	I	C
F		D	C	SD		N
S	■		C	SD		N
S	■		C	SD		N
M	*	I	N	D	C	I
Tu		I	N	D	C	L
W	*	I	N	D	C	D
Th	*	I	N	D	C	D
F	AL	N			C	D
S		I	N		C	
S		I	N		C	
M		I	N	D	C	C
Tu		I	N	L	C	D
W	*	I	D	N	C	D
Th		I	D	N	C	C
F	AL	I	D	N	D	C
S		I		N	SD	C
S		I		N	SD	C
M		C	I		N	SD
Tu		C	I	L	N	SD
W		C	I	D	N	SD
Th		C	AL	D	N	
F		C	I		N	
S		C	I		N	N
S		C	I		N	
M			C	I	D	N
Tu		D	C	I	D	N
W		D	C	AL	D	N
Th		D	C	I		N
F			C	I	D	N
S			C	I		N
S			C	I		N

C = First On Call from 8.30 a.m. to 6.30 p.m. Go to the hospital first to do postnatal checks on women in hospital, then go home unless called. Second On Call from 6.30 p.m to 8.30 a.m.

N = Second On Call at home from 8.30 a.m. to 6.30 p.m. (only to be called if needed urgently). First On Call from 6.30 p.m. to 8.30 a.m.

D = Community work (antenatal and postnatal) 8.30 a.m. to 4.30 p.m. approx.

L = Help D with Antenatal Clinic, postnatals and evening clinic

D* = Automatically allocated as another day off if you worked your last night and lost your day off

* = Meetings

Acknowledgement to Bessborough Street Team

EXAMPLE OFF DUTY

Week 1

	M	T	W	Th	F	S	S
Pam	On Call			C*	C	DO	DO
Kelly	H	O	L	I	D	A	Y
Caroline	H	H	DO	DO	H	On Call	DO
Hazel	C*	C*	*C*	H	H	DO	DO
Ann (Bank)			H	OC			H&C

Week 2

	M	T	W	Th	F	S	S
Pam	On Call		DO	C*	DO	DO	H&C
Kelly	H	H	DO	DO	H	On Call	DO
Caroline	C*	C*	*C*	H	H	DO	DO
Hazel	H	O	L	I	D	A	Y
Ann (Bank)			H	OC		H&C	

Week 1

	M	T	W	Th	F	S	S
Pam	H	H	H	H	H&C	DO	DO
Kelly	C	DO	DO	DO	On Call		C
Caroline	C*	C*	*C*	DO	DO	DO	DO
Hazel	On Call			C*	H&C	H	OC
Ann (Bank)							

Week 2

	M	T	W	Th	F	S	S
Pam	H	O	L	I	D	A	Y
Kelly	C*	H	H	H	C	H&C	DO
Caroline		C*	DO	C*	C	H&C	H&C
Hazel	H	On Call	DO	DO	DO	On Call	H&C
Ann (Bank)		*C*		OC			

CODE:
C = Community
H = Hospital Cover
* = Clinics or Classes
DO = Day Off
OC = On Call

Meetings: Monday mornings
9.15 a.m. Chamberlen

West Essex Health Authority Off Duty Rota – September 1992
Meyer Practice, Harlow

	T	W	Th	F	S	S	M	T	W	Th	F	S	S	M	T	W	Th	F	S	S	M	T	W	Th	F	S	S	M	T	W	Th
	1	2	3	4	5	6	7	8	9	10	11	12	13	14	15	16	17	18	19	20	21	22	23	24	25	26	27	28	29	30	31
Miss Seers	S		X		LW	O	S	X	O	S		X	X	O	S	LW	X	LW	O	S		X		LW		X	X		LW	O	
Mrs Mulvey	X	X	X	O	S	LW		X		X	X	X	X	X	X	X	X	O	S	O	S	X	X	X	X	X	X	X	X	X	
Mrs Ayres	X		X	X	X	X	X	X	X	X	O	S	O	S	X		X	X	X	X	X	S	X	X	AL	AL	AL	LW	X		
Miss Westall	X	LW	O	S	X	X	AL	AL	AL	X	AL	AL	AL	AL	X	AL	AL	AL	X	X	O	S	LW	X	O	S	LW	SD	X	SD	
Mrs Cooper	LW	O	S					S	X	LW	AL	X	X		LW	O	S	X	LW	AL	LW		X	O		S	X	AL	AL	AL	
Miss Kessie		X		LW	O	X	O	S		X	X	LW	LW			O	O	S	X	X	O	O	S		X	LW	O	S	S		
Mrs H/Moore	AL	AL	AL	X	AL	AL	X	LW	LW		S	X	X	LW	O	S		X	LW	LW	X		O	S	LW	X	X	O	S	S	
Mrs Bawn	O	S	LW	X	X	X	LW	O	S	X	LW	O	S	X	X	S	LW		X	X	LW	X		X		O	S	X	O	S	

Key:

Blank space	= On Duty 8.00 a.m. – 5 p.m.
ON	= On Call 5 p.m. – 8 a.m.
D	= Day Off
AL	= Annual Leave
H	= On Duty at PAH
PB & PL	= Bank Holiday ent.
C	= Course
SD	= Study Day
1/2	= On Duty 8.00 a.m. – 1.30 p.m.

Discharges:

Mon. – Fri. 8.30 a.m. – 4 p.m.
Harlow 444455 – Ext. 2491

Sat. – Sun. and late discharges contact On
Call Midwife at home

Oxford Team – T/MID 2

Nov. '91 / Dec

	3	4	5	6	7	8	9	10	11	12	13	14	15	16	17	18	19	20	21	22	23	24	25	26	27	28	29	30	1	2	3	4	5	6	7
	S	M	T	W	Th	F	S	S	M	T	W	Th	F	S	S	M	T	W	Th	F	S	S	M	T	W	Th	F	S	S	M	T	W	Th	F	S
HM	X	P	P	P	Th	F	X	X	M	T	AL	AL	F	X	X	P	P	P	Th	O	S	P	P	P	P	X	X	X	S	X			AL		X
LR		X	X	P	X	O	X	X	O		AL	AL	X	X	X	O	T	Th	W	X	O		X	O	X	X	X	X	X	X	X	O		X	X
RW	X			X	X		X	X	PL	O	X	O	X	X	X	O		X	X	X	X	X	O		X	O	X	X	O	X	O	X	O	X	X
HB		O	O		X	X	X	X	PL	PL		X	X	O	O	PL	X	X	O	X	X	X	O		X	X			X			X	X		
AS	X	X	X	X	X	X	X	O	X	X	O		X	X	X	X	X	AL	X	X	X	O	PL	X	O	X	X	X	X	O	X	O		X	O
HT	O	O		O	O	X	O	X	X	X	X	X	O	SD	X	PL	O				X		X	X	X	X	O	O				X	X	X	X
CB	X	4	4	4	4	3	3	3	4	4	3	3	3	3	3	3	3	4	3	3	3	3	4	4	3	4	4	3	3	4	4	4	4	3	3

Dec. '91 / Jan '92

	8	9	10	11	12	13	14	15	16	17	18	19	20	21	22	23	24	25	26	27	28	29	30	31	1	2	3	4	5	6	7	8	9	10	11
	S	M	T	W	Th	F	S	S	M	T	W	Th	F	S	S	M	T	W	Th	F	S	S	M	T	W	Th	F	S	S	M	T	W	Th	F	S
HM	X	X	P	P	X	X	O	X	P	P	P	X	X	O	S	M	X	O	O	X	X	X			X	X		X	X	M		AL	X		X
LR	X	P	P	O	O	X	O	X	P	P	P	X	X	O	O	O	X	O	X	X	O	X		O	X	X	X	X	X	O	X	X	X	O	X
RW	O	SD	X	X	X	X	X	X	O		AL		AL	X	X	X	X	X	X	X	X	X	X	X	X	O	X	X	O	X	X	O	X	X	X
HB	X	PL	X	O	X	O	X	X	X	O	O	X	X	X	X	O	X	X	X	X	X	O	O	X	X	X	X	X	O	X	X	X	X	X	X
AS	O		X	X	X	O	X	X	PL	X	X	X	X	X	X	X	X	X	X	X	X	O	X	X	O	O	O	O	X	X	X	X	O	X	X
HT	X	PL	X	X	X	X	X	O		O	X	O	O	O	X		AL	AL			X	X	X	X	X	X	X	X	X	X	O	X	X	X	O
CB	S	3	4	3	4	4	3	3	3	4	3	4	3	4	3	3	3	3	3	3	3	3	3	3	3	3	3	3	3	3	3	3	4	3	3

SD = Study day
P = Polytechnic
O = On Call 8 a.m – 8 a.m
□ = Normal working only
X = Day off

Australian Birth Centre

GRADE/YEAR	Grade 1	Grade 2	Grade 3	Grade 4	Grade 5	Grade 6
S						
M	TED		N	E	E	L
Tu	L		N	L	E	E
W	L	TED	N	E	E	L
Th	E	L	N	E	L	
F	E	L	TED		E	N
S		E		L		N
S		L		E		N
M	E	N		L	E	L
Tu	E	N		L	L	E
W	L	N	TED	E	E	L
Th	E	N	L	E	L	
F	E		L	E		N
S		E		L		N
S		L		E		N
M		E	L		E	N
Tu						
W						
Th						
F						
S						
S						
M						

Acknowledgements Marianne Biro

Team of Six: hospital based

LINE	Sun	Mon	Tue	Wed	Thur	Fri	Sat	Sun	Mon	Tue	Wed	Thur	Fri	Sat
Abigail	1	x	x	x	Day	Day	x	Night	Night	x	x	x	x	Day	Day
Barbara	2	Day	x	Night	Night	x	Day	Day	x	Day	Day	A/N	A/N	x	x
Colleen	3	x	A/N	A/N	A/N	x	x	x	x	A/N	A/N	A/N	A/N	A/N	x
Daphne	4	x	Day	Day	x	x	Night	Night	x	Day	Day	x	x	Day	Day
Eva	5	Night	Night	x	x	x	Day	Day	x	Night	Night	x	Night	Night	x
Frances	Senior Sister: Filling in when necessary

LINE	Sun	Mon	Tue	Wed	Thur	Fri	Sat	Sun	Mon	Tue	Wed	Thur	Fri	Sat
Eva	1	x	x	x	Day	Day	x	Night	Night	x	x	x	x	Day	Day
Abigail	2	Day	x	Night	Night	x	Day	Day	x	Day	Day	A/N	A/N	x	x
Barbara	3	x	A/N	A/N	A/N	x	x/A/N	x	x	A/N	A/N	A/N	A/N	A/N	x
Colleen	4	x	Day	Day	x	x	Night	Night	x	Day	Day	x	x	Day	Day
Daphne	5	Night	Night	x	x	x	Day	Day	x	Night	Night	x	Night	Night	x
Frances	Senior Sister: Filling in when necessary

Next Rota will be Daphne – Eva – Abigail – Barbara – Colleen
then Colleen – Daphne – Eva – Abigail – Barbara
then Barbara – Colleen – Daphne – Eva – Abigail

Continuity through antenatal period and labour and delivery. No postnatal care included

A/N = working for 9 hours in Antenatal Clinic
X = Day off
Day = Available from 08.00 to 21.00 for women in labour in delivery suite; otherwise 8 hours in Antenatal Clinic
Night = On duty from 21.00 to 08.00 in delivery suite. Probably able to look after 250 women a year.

Otago Midwives Section, Dunedin, New Zealand

	M	T	W	T	F	S	S		M	T	W	T	F	S	S		M	T	W	T	F	S	S
A	A/N	P/N	X	X	P/N	X	X^O/R		N	N	N	X	X	X	D		A/N	A/N	D	P/N	P/N	X	X
B	X	D	P/N	D	D	D	X		P/N	P/N	P/N	P/N	P/N	X	D		X	D	X	D	N	N	N
C	D	D	D	A/N	A/N	X	X		A/N	A/N	D	A/N	A/N	X^O/R	X^O/R		D	D	N	A/N	A/N	X	D
D	N	N	N	X	X	X^O/R	D		P/N	P/N	P/N	P/N	P/N	N	N		N	N	P/N	X	X	D	X^O/R
E	P/N	X	X	N	N	N	N		D	D	D	A/N	A/N	X	D		A/N	N	D	A/N	P/N	X	X

A → original C
B → original D
C → original E
D → original A
E → original B

A → original D
B → original E
C → original A
D → original B
E → original C

Continuity-of-care Midwives Scheme Sample Roster

Assumptions: on all Mondays, Tuesdays, Thursdays and Fridays, one midwife will be required to work a shift of 8 hours carrying out ante-natal duties, one an 8-hour shift carrying out postnatal duties, one on call for 12 hours during the day time for women in labour but required to work an 8-hour shift within these 12 hours assisting the A/N or P/N midwife, and finally one "on call" for 12 hours during the night time for women in labour. Wednesdays: a P/N, a D and an N, weekends a D and an N and a 3rd midwife 'on reserve'.

Legend:

A/N, P/N and D = 8-hour shifts, flexible duties, and flexible times e.g. 07.00 hrs–15.30 hrs, 08.00 hrs–18.30 hrs, 13.00 hrs–21.30 hrs, according to need/demand/on call hours worked

D = an 8-hour shift plus 4 hours on call from 08.00 hrs to 20.00 hrs
N = 12 hours on call 20.00 hrs to 08.00 hrs
X = day off
X$^{O/R}$ = day off, but 'on reserve' in case required to assist duty midwife

Rota One: a week period – 160 official work hours

A works: 120 hours of on-duty shift work
56 hours 'on call'
B works: 104 hours of on duty shift work
84 hours 'on call'
C works: 112 hours of on duty shift work
96 hours 'on call'
D works: 88 hours of on duty shift work
104 hours 'on call'
E works: 88 hours of on duty shift work
108 hours on call

Acknowledgements Sally Pairman

8

Hospital teams

Most midwives in the United Kingdom work in hospital and most women have their babies in hospital. Within many Units in the United Kingdom Team Schemes are being set up or tried. It would appear that there are several motives for setting up Teams.

First, Team Schemes may be set up because there is a genuine attempt to enable women to get to know their midwives better and to form a relationship with them. Secondly, Team Schemes may be set up in an attempt to utilise staff more effectively and to move away from the scenario of six midwives on the Labour Ward sitting and watching television while the midwives in the Postnatal Ward are flying around with too much to do. Thirdly, setting up a Hospital Team Scheme may be in response to pressures, either from women, midwives or the Unit General Manager – the total effect may be purely cosmetic, no change in working practices, no change in working hours, no greater intimacy between women and midwives. All the Schemes set up so far appear to enable midwives to relate to each other better and to get to know each other better. This in itself may have a beneficial effect.

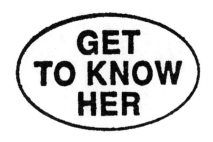

With Teams set up in hospitals, usually the midwives are unwilling or unable to be on call, they wish to work the shift patterns that they work at present. The differing philosophies of greater continuity of care for women and for more efficient utilisation of staff do not always automatically coincide and just because midwives are grouped into Teams does not ever mean that women necessarily get to know a midwife through their pregnancy who will then care for them during labour, and this is what women are asking us for and have done over many years.

In Riverside Health Authority from 1990 an intention was made for increasing continuity of carer for women within the hospital. Teams of midwives were set up – it ended up with staff being more efficiently allocated and with midwives getting to know each other better, but it is doubtful whether the amount of continuity for women increased.

To initiate change within a hospital needs to be done with the same preparation as carried out when any changes are being contemplated. First, being employed as the consultant to plan and implement the change I initially roamed around the Hospital and got to know all the midwives. I got to know all their names, their faces, I tried to find out what made them tick, what their family circumstances were, what pressures were on them and generally tried to foster a supportive and open feeling between myself and them. I also interviewed women in the Postnatal Wards and women in the Antenatal Clinic to find out how the organization worked and how women perceived the way that they were looked after.

What I discovered was that women saw different midwives each week when they came to the Antenatal Clinic and they also had to wait for long periods. They expressed a desire to have the same person looking after them during their pregnancy and that same person looking after them during their labour. The same complaints came up in the Postnatal Ward, there was also some criticism of the attitude of some of the midwives who were on Night Duty. Conversely there was great praise for some of the midwives on Night Duty who looked after them very well when they were in labour.

I then did some presentations for all the midwives. First, to relate back to them what the women had said about the service they were receiving, and, secondly, to show them acetates photocopied from the notes. The acetates showed only the signatures and the comments from women's Antenatal Clinic visits, and this was really enough to convince any midwife that women did not receive continuity of carer and that they really did see a different person every time they came to the Antenatal Clinic. I would always encourage midwives to look in the women's notes in their wards and to note how many different midwives and doctors they see.

Following the presentations and the publication of a report on the survey I had done in the Hospital, Action Group meetings were set up. These occurred every fortnight and during the Action Group meetings we first of all got to know each other and then talked through ways to develop the working practices within the hospital which would improve continuity of carer for women and would enable us to set up Teams.

It was exceedingly difficult for midwives to get to know each other, perhaps because during the time the midwives had been nurses they had been encouraged not to get involved with their patients or perhaps because the midwives saw themselves as needing to be rather invincible, they were certainly unwilling to show the more vulnerable sides of themselves to others. Whatever the reason midwives seem to keep themselves to themselves and find it difficult to share their problems or their different life events with anybody except a very few, very close friends.

It always seems to me that unless we know each other well it is very difficult for us to make allowances for each other or even to become fond of each other. The more we are able to get to know other human beings the more we can understand what makes them tick and what drives them, and it is very important that we share details of our lives with each other because it makes it much easier for us to be understanding of each other and caring of each other.

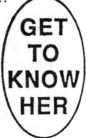

GET TO KNOW HER

Different ways of helping people to get to know each other are discussed in Chapter 9. As humans get to know each other better they are more motivated to cooperate with each other more easily and to make allowances for each other. It would appear that it is more difficult to initiate change within a Hospital than it is in the Community because of several factors. First, in the Hospital, the work of the midwife has been fragmented and split up for many years so there are midwives who have been in the Labour Ward for 7, 10 or 15 years who function brilliantly within the Labour Ward but have no idea of how to book a woman, how to provide antenatal care, how to provide postnatal care, how to help with breastfeeding or even how to discharge a woman on the computer.

Likewise there are midwives who have worked in the Antenatal Clinic for years and years, who are terrified at the thought of going into the Labour Ward, as are midwives who work in the Postnatal Ward. These midwives have developed their skill in one area of care during childbirth but it is at the cost of other areas.

Another problem about changing the way that people in Hospital work is that frequently the midwives in a Hospital have been working the same shifts and in the same way for many years, such as the midwife who always does Tuesday and Thursday nights and no others, or the midwife who does Friday and Saturday nights and no others. There is often no need to change the way they work but if it is seen as necessary it can cause great problems and in fact at the West London Hospital when trying to initiate the Teams, despite dozens of opportunities of talking through the changes and to contribute to the changes, and despite meetings being held at times which were convenient for night staff, and despite the Consultant having gone in to meet the night staff on many different occasions, the midwives on night duty took out a grievance which lasted for a year and held up the initiation of the Hospital Teams for all that period.

Maybe with greater consultation this could have been avoided, but it is difficult to see how greater consultation could have been achieved or how the grievance could have been avoided considering all the work done with midwives on night duty prior to them taking out a grievance.

Changing working practices makes passions rise, many people feel very threatened and distressed by changes in their working arrangements.

Continuity of carer or more efficient deployment of staff?

Most of the Hospital Team schemes that I have been privy to seem to enable the staff to be deployed in a more efficient manner and often enable the midwives to get to know each other better as well. This probably has benefits for the women. If you are being looked after by midwives who know and like each other it is probably more pleasant than being looked after by midwives who do not know each other very well, but as far as I can see this is the only benefit which is gained from most Hospital Team Schemes.

North Middlesex and the West London Hospital

The schemes based at the North Middlesex and West London Hospitals are similar, they are both Consultant based so that each Team includes a Consultant Obstetrician in the Team and each Team's base is a Postnatal Ward. When it is their Consultant's Antenatal Clinic two or three of the midwives from the Team go to the Antenatal Clinic and take part in order to hold antenatal consultations and checks and to see and get to know the women from their Team. The overall running of the Clinic is performed by a Health Care Assistant (at the West London Hospital). The midwives provide Parentcraft Classes and this enables them to get to know quite a few of the women, but it is not usually a very involved type of relationship.

When the woman goes into labour she rings up the Postnatal Ward rather than the Labour Ward and speaks to one of 'her' midwives, the woman comes into the Hospital when it is appropriate and is assessed either on the Postnatal Ward or the Labour Ward. She is then looked after by a midwife from 'her' Team.

Postnatally she is looked after by the same group of midwives in the Postnatal Ward. There are advantages and disadvantages to this type of scheme:

- The greatest disadvantage is that if the woman is looked after in labour by a midwife she knows it is quite by chance.
- The advantages are that the woman MAY be looked after in labour by a midwife she knows.
- She is looked after postnatally by midwives she has got to know beforehand.
- The staff are deployed more efficiently.
- Midwives get to know each other better and enjoy better working relationships.

From the survey reported in Chapter 3 it can be seen that the midwives had greater job satisfaction working in the Hospital Teams than they had before the setting up of the Teams.

More efficient deployment of staff comes from the fact that instead of the Labour Ward, Antenatal Clinic and Postnatal Clinic being staffed separately, all the staff are based on the Postnatal Ward and they are then allocated to the area where women need them to be.

The allocation of the staff to different areas may be done in advance so that a midwife may know that she is going to be in the Antenatal Clinic on Wednesday afternoon and Friday morning, and for the rest of the week she is going to be in the Postnatal Ward except for when she is called to the Labour Ward because a woman from her team is in labour. At the North Middlesex Hospital this is always done in advance so the midwife knows when she is going to be in the Delivery Suite as well. At the West London Hospital a small sign on the off duty indicates that this is the day when that specific midwife will be in the Labour Ward if a woman calls her, but until that happens she works on the Postnatal Ward. Here a further disadvantage reveals itself, if the midwife is called to a woman in labour she is often in the middle of postnatal care to a group of women and has to abruptly leave the women she is looking after.

At the West London Hospital there is a co-ordinator of each Team who is on duty each day (the co-ordinator is the most senior midwife from that Team who is on duty that day). When the co-ordinator comes on duty she goes to the Labour Ward to see if any of the women from her Team are in labour and then she allocates whoever is to go from the Postnatal Ward to look after that woman (or women). The advantage is that midwives are where the women need them to be and are not twiddling their thumbs in the Labour Ward waiting for something to happen or cleaning cupboards. On the other hand midwives find it quite disorientating, especially at first, to keep being moved, but as time goes by they find it more and more easy and instead of feeling that they are working on Ward Six and that is 'their' ward, they begin to feel that they work in that Hospital and they enjoy the development of their allround skills.

Leicester Home from Home Unit

In 1988 three rooms were opened within Leicester Royal Infirmary's Delivery Suite. These three rooms looked like normal bedrooms, they had normal beds as would be found in anybody's bedroom, the floors were carpetted, there were curtains, bedspreads and rocking chairs and all of the equipment that is usually found in a Hospital Labour Ward was removed. Women using these rooms could not have epidurals, nor could they have continuous fetal heart monitoring, they were treated as if they were having a home birth. Fetal monitoring was to take place with a Pinards stethoscope and women were enabled and encouraged to take up any position that they wanted to.

Originally there was one Team of eight midwives, and it was presumed that they would be able to look after 1200 women a year with at least 400 of those women being transferred during pregnancy to more intensive medical supervision, it was expected that the eight midwives would then look after 800 women a year. There are now two teams of 11 WTE midwives and between them they do 1109 deliveries. Seventy per cent of bookings are done in the woman's home by a Community Midwife who uses a categorisation form which enables a woman to be categorised as being low risk, high risk or according to her own choice.

Women in Leicester Health Authority can either have their baby at home or they can take part in a GP scheme, in which 14 GPs are involved, or they can be looked after in the Home from Home scheme, which is run by midwives who are based in the

Labour and Delivery Suite and practise in the Home from Home rooms. Women get to know the Home from Home midwives by attending a clinic with them three times during their pregnancy. They attend this clinic at 26, 36 and 41 weeks if they get to that stage. When a woman goes into labour she rings the Home from Home Unit and speaks to one of the Home from Home midwives. She comes into hospital bringing with her whoever she wishes to, her husband, her mother, her next door neighbour, her children, everybody is welcome. During labour she is able to eat a light diet, she is encouraged to move about, she is encouraged to have a bath.

Further studies have shown that the job satisfaction of midwives in the Home from Home Unit is exceedingly high and recruitment and retention has been increased. The Home from Home midwives have their own Postnatal Ward of 26 beds, so the woman is guaranteed postnatal care by the midwife who delivered her the previous day. Many women have a 6-hour discharge when they are discharged straight from the Home from Home rooms. The midwives are helped by five support workers who work mostly in the Postnatal Ward. Soon to be published is the data which shows that the women in the Home from Home Unit have much the same outcomes as women in the main Unit. Women appear to find the homely atmosphere very conducive to a pleasant birth experience and the possibility of having a midwife that they know increases their pleasure.

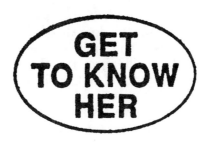

GET TO KNOW HER

9

Team building

In order to work together as effectively as possible, it is essential that midwives working in a Team learn to trust each other and get to know each other. There are different ways of helping midwives to do this and what I hope to present to you in this chapter is a potpourri of ideas so that you can look at different ways to help midwives to get to know each other better.

Change is incredibly painful, even change which is welcome is disorientating and difficult and very upsetting for those people going through it. Before the changes the midwife knows where she is working, how she is working, what time she will be off duty, what she will be doing at 10 o'clock, what she needs to do in specific situations, what she should not do in specific situations, where everything is kept for her to carry out her job, everything is laid out and easy.

Following change the midwife is not sure where she should be, how she should be reacting, who her friends are, what time she is off duty, where she should be at this moment, where she should be in a quarter of an hour's time, what she should do when she has got nothing to do. All of this involves great disorientation and distress and midwives need to be prepared for this otherwise they will reject the change as being too painful to contemplate and will not realise that this is just a temporary adjunct to that change.

How do we get people to work with each other as a Team, so that they can support each other through this difficult time, and then having accomplished the changes, they can continue to support and help each other? The first and most important facet of supporting each other is that your Team members need to meet each other and talk with each other, there is no other way of getting to know people than actually by face to face discussion and listening.

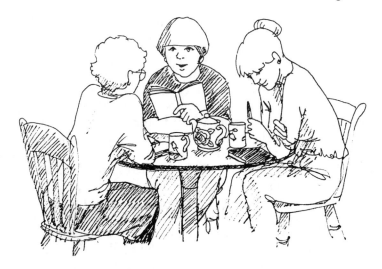

Because midwives find it difficult and threatening to reveal details of themselves to each other they will do anything in their power to avoid meeting with each other, so whatever time the meeting is proposed for it will be inconvenient for a great many of the midwives, whatever venue is chosen will be inconvenient for many of the midwives. It is exceedingly difficult to get midwives together just to talk to each other. They will feign that it is unimportant or that they know each other already, all these excuses have to be ignored and meetings need to be made to start at a time when people cannot easily get out of them, 8 a.m. is quite a good time, before the telephone begins to ring and before anyone begins to start the day's work.

Feeling welcomed

Midwives need to be made welcome at their meeting and it can be very cheering to be greeted with a cup of coffee or a cup of tea and maybe a few croissants or some toast at 8 a.m., and if midwives know that they are going to be looked after in this way it makes it easier for them to come to the meeting. This, of course, depends upon the resources available to the person who is trying to build the Team.

Right at the beginning the Team will not know each other at all and it is important that they should be meeting with those who they are going to be working closely with, such as, Health Visitors, or the Receptionist in their Clinic or the Caretaker, and if all these people can be included in the first few meetings that the Team has, this can enable them to feel part of the project and to feel warmly towards the Team members. The meeting needs to be started with everyone in the room telling everybody else what their names are and something about themselves. 'The something about themselves' needs to be non-threatening and not very personal, so it can be along the lines of how they got here this morning: "My name is Mary Robinson and I travelled here today from Barnes and I came on the No. 48 bus and I needed to leave at 7.05 a.m. to get here on time", or it can be along the lines of their hobby "I'm Joan and what I like to do when I'm off duty is bread making", or "I'm Vinolia and what is really having fun for me is to go to Stringfellows and to dance until the early hours". Choose topics which are non-invasive and non-threatening, whatever you choose helps people to realise how their colleagues tick, or what travelling difficulties, or what interests others members of the Team have.

The first workshops for Team building should last no more than half a day and probably a couple of hours is enough. Eventually the group needs to spend time visualising the way in which it will be working when the new system starts. The group can be split up into smaller groups of three and four people and they can be asked to describe how they see a typical day, or how they would expect to be working once the new scheme starts. The Caretaker can be given an opportunity to say how it is going to affect him. The Receptionist needs to know who is coming to the front door and where they will need to be directed to. Don't forget the Medical Records Staff who will need to know the implications of the new scheme as far as medical records are concerned. Everybody who can be inveigled into coming to this meeting should do so.

Several meetings/workshops should be set up before a new Scheme starts so that everybody is able to get to know each other but also so that the participants in the Scheme can work through in their minds how they will be working and they can begin to visualise how that work will be when they start.

Eventually, probably after the first couple of workshops, it needs to be only the Midwife Team who need to work together, but it must be remembered that the other people who are affected by the Team, such as Caretakers, Medical Records Staff, etc., need to be invited to these meetings from time to time, probably every 2–3 months, so that they can report back any problems or difficulties that they are having, and working practices can be adjusted accordingly.

Weekly meetings

In order to get to know each other the Team must meet each other face to face, and in order to keep pace with the ever-changing world that they are working in, midwives need to meet at least weekly. The weekly meetings need to be set at a time and in a place that is convenient for most people and these should take place even if very few people turn up to them. On the other hand, if very few people turn up to them those who have not attended need to be persuaded/cajoled into coming and it needs to be stressed how important it is for a Team to become a Team and that this will only happen if these people turn up to the meetings. It needs to be agreed that if decisions are taken at the Team meeting then these decisions are binding on all other members of the Team, whether they are present or not, which often gives an incentive for other members to turn up because they want to have a say in how the Team works.

In order for the Team to get to know each other they need, each time, to reiterate their names. This may sound ridiculous and probably is if there are only five or six people in the Team, but it can take quite a while for people to get to know each others' names, and if staff changes it is surprising how few people know each others' names. It is enormously embarrassing to have forgotten someone's name – especially someone you are 'supposed' to know. Midwives can go around the room and say what their names are, and then they can say other things which are non-threatening to them so that they can get to know each other. They can say such things as 'something bad and something good that has happened in my life since we last met each other', for instance: "My name is Jodie and the bad thing that has happened to me in the last week is that my car broke down

last Wednesday and I have had to borrow a car from the pool
and when I got it it was really smokey and disgusting. The good
thing that has happened to me is that my son has really settled
down well at his nursery and seems to be enjoying it and has
stopped crying every time I leave him in the morning, so it is
much easier for me to leave every day."

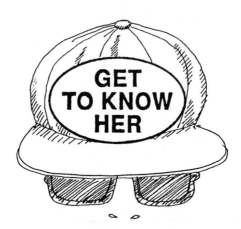

The midwives can say their name and what they would be
doing if it was their day off today and this gives an insight as to
whether people are doing dozens of domestic chores on their
day off, or whether they are looking after themselves by having
a massage or a swim, or whether they are studying or all the
other things that midwives can be doing. Midwives can go
around the room and say what their name is and what they
would do if they were to win half a million pounds in a
competition, how they would spend their life and whether they
would still be working as midwives.
    An interesting subject is to ask each person to say what their
name is and then to say something that is completely unique
about them in this room – and if it is not unique and someone
else shares the same characteristic, they must challenge the first
person who must then think of another facet which is totally
unique. For instance, "I'm Gloria and I'm the only person in the
room who is pregnant", "I'm Rebecca and I'm the only person
in this room who took their dog out for a walk at 7 o'clock this
morning".

Other ways of getting to know each other better are by saying one's name and what is special about your name, or what you like about your name, or why you are called that name – "I'm called Barbara after my Grandma" (Houston, 1984). Midwives can go around the room and say what gives them most pleasure in their life or what gives them the greatest fun. As the group develops the midwives can go around the room and say the most interesting thing they have learned during the last week, and this can encourage them to bring snippets from the newspaper or from medical and nursing journals which can add to the knowledge in the group.

Agenda and meetings book

There should be a book in which the weekly meetings are written down. An agenda should be written on one side of the page and this can be added to by anybody, and on the right hand side of the book the actions from that agenda should be dealt with, so that peoople can look back through the book and recognise when they decided on certain things and see what was agreed at the time. They can also look at last week's agenda before this week's meeting and quickly do the things they were supposed to do before the meeting starts or the day before. "I wrote to Jeremy, but I only posted it this morning so I haven't got a reply yet".

Treats

Other ways of getting to know each other are by going away together, either for a day or for longer, and by going out to enjoy oneself. The Christmas outing is exceedingly important, so probably is the Summer outing, the Easter outing and any other outings one can think of. Spending time together outside work is very important. For the group to feel cherished and pampered such experiences as having a manicurist to manicure the nails of the whole group can be very therapeutic, as can having someone just to massage everybody's shoulders, people who are good at massaging shoulders or feet can do that for the rest of the group and this can be extremely pleasant.

In *Nursing Times* of 19 June 1991 Marie Manthey, President of Creative Nursing Management, Minneapolis, USA quotes a charter for co-workers which could be useful to put up and to try to adhere to:

STATEMENT OF COMMITMENT TO CO-WORKERS

As your co-worker with a shared goal of providing excellent nursing care to our patients, I commit the following:

I will accept responsibility for establishing and maintaining healthy interpersonal relationships with you and every member of this staff. I will talk to you promptly if I am having a problem with you. The only time I will discuss it with another person is when I need advice or help in deciding how to communicate with you appropriately.

I will establish and maintain a relationship of functional trust with you and every member of this staff. My relationships with each of you will be equally respectful, regardless of job titles or levels of educational preparation.

I will not engage in the '3B's' (bickering, back-biting and bitching) and will ask you not to as well.

I will not complain about another team member and ask you not to as well. If I hear you doing so I will ask you to talk to that person.

I will accept you as you are today, forgiving past problems, and ask you to do the same with me.

I will be committed to finding solutions to problems, rather than complaining about them or blaming someone, and ask you to do the same.

I will affirm your contribution to quality patient care.

I will remember that neither of us is perfect, and that human errors are opportunities not for shame or guilt but for forgiveness and growth.

Physical contact

Touching each other makes people feel closer, and from our experience of young children and their needs it would appear that human beings have a natural need to be touched, stroked and hugged. Because of our natural reserve we find it difficult to hug and stroke one another, especially when we are females together, but as love grows between a team of midwives often this develops naturally with people patting and stroking each other, or hugging each other when they meet or say goodbye.

One way of touching each other in a non-threatening way is to shake each others' hands when meeting or to make a point of always patting each member of the team when you meet them. Some midwives will find this very easy to do, others will find it very difficult, the feelings about this should be explored within the group because some people may feel invaded if they are being patted by other people, whereas other people will feel very accepted and pleased at being touched by other human beings. As midwives we often touch women, sometimes we are not so happy about people touching us. This is an aspect of our practice that we should be aware of.

What are we saying about our own perceptions and about our own personalities if we feel that it is acceptable to touch other people but we do not feel it is acceptable for them to touch us?

There are some games one can use to help people touch each other in an unthreatening way and also to learn to trust each other. One good game is for one person to be blindfolded and the other person leads them about so that the person who is blindfolded has to give the person who is leading them their complete trust. Another exercise is for the group to stand in a circle all facing in the same direction, either clockwise or anticlockwise, and then the person who is initiating the exercise can describe a rainstorm and each person makes a rainstorm on the person in front on their shoulders and back. The rainstorm starts quite gently, pitter-patter, pitter-patter, as the person feels the pitter-pattering of the fingers of the person behind her on her back, the rainstorm starts with gentle and slow pitter-patters and then begins to speed up as the drops of rain become bigger and bigger, and wetter and wetter. The storm continues and the raindrops begin to fall faster and faster so that they are soaking the person's head, shoulders and back, and it goes faster and faster until the storm is beginning to pass and the pitter-patter of the rain becomes slower and slower until it finally drops away. To touch people on their back and shoulders is non-threatening and non-sexual and is acceptable to most people.

One lovely way of touching, which is favoured by the Association of Radical Midwives, is what is called a belly laugh. One person lies down and the next person lies down using the tummy of the first person lying down as her pillow, the next person lies down and puts her head on the second person and so on until everybody in the room is lying with their head on somebody's tummy. Then the group just waits and eventually somebody will start to laugh and the feeling of amusement and delight this brings as one's head is wobbled up and down by somebody's tummy when they are laughing is such fun that eventually everybody begins to laugh and it is an exceedingly delightful exercise, but it needs a degree of trust in the other people and a degree of cleanliness of the floor in the room that you are doing this in.

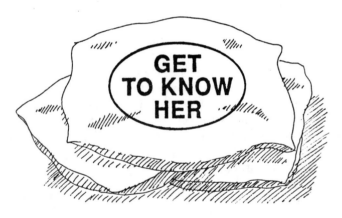

Looking ahead

During Team meetings it is especially important for members of the Team to look ahead – to vision where they are planning to go in the future. Just as individuals have personal goals, "I want to own my own place by 1999", or "I want to have a baby by 1997", or "By the time I am 37 I intend to be fluent in French", so does a Team or Unit need to know where it is aiming to go.

If a Team does not look towards the future what it does now will become static and the Team will become static and will stop growing and developing. So the Team needs to look ahead:

- "What we would like to be doing in 5 years time."
- "How we see the Team developing in the next 5 years."
- "Where we see the Team functioning in the next 5 years."
- "What we envisage the midwives doing in the next 5 years."
- "How we can improve our practice in the next 5 years."
- "How can we make our service more responsive to women in the next 5 years."
- "What sort of research we aim to have done in the next 5 years."

Working in a Team can be a source of great growth and joy for those midwives who are members of it, learning and knowledge grow as women become more assertive and ask you more complicated questions during the time you are looking after them – Team colleagues challenge your practice so you have to be able to justify it by decent research, it's no good saying "I always do it this way", every action needs to be thought through and justified – challenging, but so exciting!

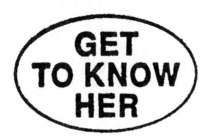

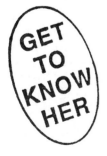

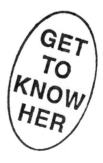

10

Disadvantages and hurdles

The deep depression which follows the setting up of a continuity of carer scheme has already been mentioned. It is common for midwives setting out on a new way of working to feel very, very enthusiastic during the first few days of their exciting new venture. This excitement quickly gives way to feelings of isolation, disorientation and deep depression. There are many reasons for this. First, the midwife has left the known environment of either the ward or the community in which she worked before. Before the start of the scheme she knew what time she would be off duty, when specific things were done each day, who her friends were, how the ward routine worked, where the pathology forms were kept, how to order drugs for the drug cupboard, the list goes on and on. When a new scheme starts everybody has to learn right from the beginning how to run it and what happens within it.

When Teams are set up in the Community the most basic actions cause enormous work and effort. A woman needs to be visited in Algarve Road, it's her first day postnatally, the midwives do not know where Algarve Road is. When they reach Algarve Road they find that it is a one-way street and they have approached from the wrong end, and anyway the numbers are not in the normal numbering and they cannot find the house they need. When it is not only Algarve Road, but Fitzimmons Street, Acre Lane and Johnsons Mews, all of which have to be looked up on the map and all of which have to be found for the very first time, work becomes exceedingly tiring. If the number of visits which have to be done are eight or ten, the midwife arrives home totally exhausted, and also totally muddled as to where she has been and which woman she saw in each house or flat.

If only one Scheme has been set up as in a Pilot Scheme the midwives have nobody to turn to but each other, when discovering that they are disorientated and depressed. Often they feel that they cannot say this to each other because it seems almost shameful that they feel so depressed when they are taking part in something that they have been wanting to take part in for some time. If there is more than one Team and the Team members can get together they will find with great delight that other members will feel the same and that other Team members have grumpier caretakers in their Health Authority Building, or even less cooperative GPs, or even more one-way systems, or have had their cars clamped even more times, and this can be very helpful to midwives and the value of joint Team meetings cannot be overemphasised.

One of the most stressful manifestations of working in a situation providing continuity of care is being on call. Many midwives find it very difficult to sleep when they are on call initially, all the time they think they might be called and they are afraid of missing the bleep signal if they are deeply asleep, and again they are afraid of being woken out of sleep once they are deeply asleep. Many midwives find it extremely hard that they cannot drink any alcohol nor can they go out to the theatre just in case they are called. With the advent of long range bleepers and especially message pagers, the problem of being on call can almost be eliminated. First, the midwife can travel outside her home, secure in the knowledge that she will be able to be contacted if she goes out to visit friends or to the theatre.

The women can be trained that when they leave a message with bleep control they give details of the reason why they have bleeped and also the telephone number on which they can be contacted. So for instance instead of getting a call "please ring 071 498 0698", the midwife will receive calls which say "Dear Joan, It's Mary Robinson here. Just to let you know that I have had a show but I am not having any contractions yet. I thought you would like to know. I'm on 081 229 0613 and I will bleep you again if anything more exciting is happening". On the other hand the bleep message may be "Fiona Richard here. Can I change my antenatal appointment that is arranged for 11 a.m.

tomorrow because I have to go to my daughter's school to go and see her teacher? I could make it on Wednesday or Friday at any time during the day if that would be convenient for you. With love Fiona 071 283 4567".

When women have been encouraged to give the reason for their message, being on call for the midwife is much less stressful. The midwife knows that she will be forewarned when receiving a message from a woman, she knows whether she needs to respond immediately or when the theatre has finished, or whether she can leave it until the morning.

On call all the time

Often, when midwives are on call or working in a way which provides continuity of care, they feel as if they are on duty all the time. Often this is self-induced in that the majority of midwives working in Teams appear to leave their bleeps on all the time so that they can see what has been going on when they are off duty, often they leave the bleep on 'mute' so that it makes no noise, but they are forever looking at it to see what's going on while they are away!

The feeling of always being at work may just be part of being a professional person. Midwives are not people who work from 9 a.m. to 5 p.m. and then 'clock off' and have no further involvement or commitment, they are people who think about and care about the women they look after all the time. When they are off duty they can be discussing midwifery, or writing an article on midwifery, or reading a midwifery book, or a book about childbirth. If this means that they feel that they are never off duty they are probably right and they probably never are off duty, but often this just means that they have a great interest in their subject and they are fulfilling the role of a professional woman who needs to think through and think forward about her profession.

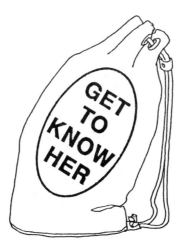

One of the ways of overcoming the stress of working in a continuity of carer scheme is for the midwives to get to know each other very well and by doing so they will become exceedingly fond of each other and will give extra support to each other. This is why it is so important to have weekly meetings with other members of the Team and so important to give something personal of each midwife, every week, at the Team meeting, otherwise it is impossible to get to know one another. Once midwives get to know each other and become 'best friends' they will quite automatically be kind and generous towards each other most of the time, and will save each other from stress when they pick it up in each other.

There is one scenario where this may not happen and this is in the case in which a Team may pick on one midwife as the scapegoat and may bully or pick on that Team member in an unkind way. This sickness in the Team needs to be addressed with professional counselling and support for the whole Team and it is very distressing for the person who is being picked on and it is also very disruptive to the whole functioning of the Team.

To work within a group of committed midwives usually means that intellectually the midwives are stimulated by each other, and because the sort of midwives who become involved in continuity of care schemes are usually highly committed midwives they will be able to offer to each other enormous advantages and specific learning opportunities because each of them will read different things and will be able to offer to the Team different things that they have learned.

Another way of overcoming the stress of being on call is for each midwife to have her own caseload of women that she has been able to get to know. If the bleep message always comes from someone she knows and is fond of it is much easier for the midwife. If as well the midwife knows exactly who she has booked each month and if the bleep goes off it has to be Mary who was due on the 8th, or Fiona who was due on the 9th or Verity who was due last month but seems to be going on for ever, it feels copeable with and manageable.

Different phases of the team

In his book *Managing Change and Making it Stick*, Roger Plant describes the phases through which an organisation goes during its development. Phase 1 is the autocratic phase when the pioneer or the founder is the driving force and the source of enthusiasm for all members. As this is an important phase in the development of all organisational change it would seem that it may be important for Teams to have a Team Leader, but the Riverside Teams have been highly successful despite not having a Team Leader and the leadership of the Team being rotated about every 6 months with varying degrees of success.

Each area and each organisation will develop its midwifery Teams in its own special way, but it is worth thinking about the advantages and disadvantages of having a Team Leader. As somebody who loves to lead and who was born organising most of my fellows I could not bear to be in a Team where I was not the leader, but having said that, I am aware that this style is not for everybody.

Plant describes Phase 2 as the bureaucratic phase where everything is spelled out and every job is described and the Team begins to work like a well-organised machine. Plant summarises this phase as:

1. Division of work in an orderly and stable fashion.
2. Systemisation of rules and procedures.

3. Establishment of hierarchy in which lower ranks are governed by higher.
4. Distribution of authority through a number of levels in a systematic manner.
5. Promotion on the basis of qualifications and experience.
6. Rules and procedures override the requirements of the situation.

Phase 3 is described by Plant as the democratic phase when people in an organisation work as Teams, with all people in the Team being respected as having a valid and equal input.

Nothing is static and Teams develop and progress and change as different members become pregnant and go off on maternity leave or retire or just get other jobs. Teams are in a constant state of flux and a desire is often expressed for everything to be 'normal and settled again'. As long as the Team keeps its weekly meetings and continues to get to know each other and care for each other, it will be able to cope with the different changes and stresses, but this must be kept an eye on because it is very easy for the Team to drift off into not having weekly meetings and into losing touch with each other.

Leon Hall in the *Leadership and Organization Development Journal* describes the importance of helping everyone in the Team to have a common vision. He points out that "Blame is largely useless and often damaging", and he suggests striving for times when "Public Celebrations" can take place, rather than "Public Executions", and that Team members and especially their managers should look out for ways of celebrating performance that demonstrates and supports the communal vision (Hall, 1991).

He describes ownership, and says that it becomes evident when people begin to talk about the vision as if it were their own. He describes a process of evaluation which necessitates asking three questions:

1. Are we achieving the vision? What is our proof?
2. Is the vision reflected in our objectives (individual and group) and our priorities?
3. Is the vision reflected in how we allocate our resources?

He goes on to describe a system of periodic review in which further questions are asked:

4. Is our current vision still relevant?
5. Do the factors which made the change imperative still exist?
6. Does some current or anticipated external change require a new or refined vision?

A disadvantage?

One of the aspects which has not been evaluated which appears to be a consequence of continuity of carer and the midwife and the woman getting to know each other, is the increased powerfulness of the midwife and the mothers. It is exceedingly difficult to evaluate this rather nebulous concept, but it was evident in the behaviour of the women in the Tooting, Know Your Midwife Scheme, that they were perceived by midwives who were not in the Know Your Midwife Scheme, as being 'bolshie'. The women, who all came from a poor area of South London, felt that they had the right to refuse to have medical students in the room with them, or the right to have their baby in the bed with them, or their right to express an opinion at a time when most people would not expect women to express an opinion.

Not only do women appear to become more powerful and, therefore, more threatening to those who are looking after them (but not to those of their carers who have actually got to know them), but so also do midwives. In Frances Evans' report on the Newcastle Community Care Project (Evans, 1987), she identifies this and the resentment it causes:

> Although there was this significant improvement in job satisfaction among community midwives, they felt that this would have been further enhanced were it not for the opposition they felt they encountered from some of the hospital medical staff. There have been several minor incidents during the life of the Project when Project midwives have taken on rather more responsibility for the patient than is usual and this has caused complaint from the medical staff. Indeed, two of the five project midwives said their main source of job dissatisfaction was that they felt some of the hospital medical staff were antagonistic towards the Project.

It is interesting to note that the Scunthorpe midwives were treated differently from the other midwives by the medical staff – enabled to practise much more autonomously.

Although there is no research evidence to either validate or invalidate this, it appears that many Doctors could find it threatening when midwives take on what they perceive to be their full role, and with the greater confidence of midwives problems can occur in the relationship with Obstetricians. Equally doctors who are confident in themselves and do not feel threatened by midwives often encourage them and can be a source of great comfort and friendship. It would be almost impossible to evaluate this because it is unlikely that doctors are going to admit to feeling threatened by midwives, but it is thought to be the basis of the closure of the Know Your Midwife Scheme in Tooting, the sabotage by GPs of a similar project proposed in Manchester and is evident from the sabotage efforts by a small group of GPs in Riverside Health Authority.

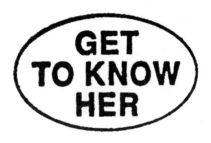

11

Use of health care assistants

In my life and work as a midwife I use many assistants, they do not have the title of Health Care Assistants, and in fact one of them has the title husband. Some of my assistants are employed, some are there because of ties of love, and they assist and help in the work of this midwife.

Husbands

My husband Giles washes my clothes, cooks my food, often makes the bed and does occasional bits of shopping. All these enable me, as a midwife, to practise more efficiently and to fulfil the role for which I have been trained. Many husbands cannot do as much as Giles does but his work is very regular and he gets home earlier than I do, and he is less tired than I am, and because he is a very fair-minded man he will often carry on and cook the supper just because he is home earlier than me.

Giles also gets the pillows out for when I do an antenatal class, and will often clear away the cups at the end. What is his reward for this? The rewards are not very tangible – he earns my gratitude and he has a sweeter-tempered wife because of his ministrations. He is also interested in birth and new families, his help at the birth of our own children was for me very important and for him, kindled an interest in childbearing that was not present before.

Girl Friday

Janet Andrews has worked with me for 5 years and she is an enormous help as a right hand woman, as she is also one of my oldest friends (we were young mothers together 27 years ago) she feels at liberty to keep me in order, to tell me when she disagrees with something I want to do, and gives me the enormous delight of working with someone I am very fond of. Not only does Janet type (and sometimes compose) letters, follows up phone calls, makes enquiries, orders goods, she also goes to the Passport Office, or does the supermarket shopping, goes to the bank, or the cash dispenser and delivers or collects urgent mail, takes the car to the car wash or acts as a chauffeur when I need to leave my car behind in the garage and generally does the jobs that I have not time to do.

There is no doubt in my mind that secretarial/administrative/supportive help is essential to busy professional midwives. This help can vary from taking the papers to the paper collecting bin and the bottles to the bottle bank, finding out how you address someone in the House of Lords to finding out what the Fax number of Downing Street is; it can vary from fixing up appointments with ultrasound, to sending off Guthrie tests, to writing letters to GPs, Obstetricians or Supervisors of Midwives. All these things take time, energy and effort and do not need a midwifery qualification to do them. Midwives are best at doing midwifery and if they employ somebody to support them they will find they can achieve far more because of that support than they can when they try to do everything on their own. They will become more productive and as they become more productive they will also become more financially viable.

It is false economy to say that one cannot afford a secretary or a helper – it is much more sensible to recognise one's skills and to realise that other people have skills in other fields and to utilise those skills.

Janet will prepare a lunch for people invited to a business meal, or will water or attend to the plants on the balcony. Janet is not called a Health Care Assistant but she certainly assists this midwife and enables her to carry out her midwifery functions efficiently and with much less stress than if she was not with me.

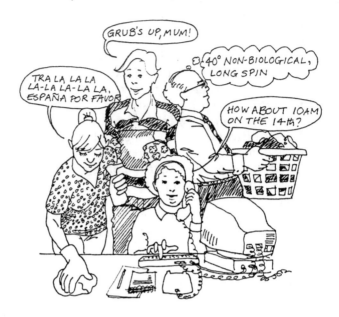

Mother's Help/Home Help

There are several different sorts of help. We employ Mother's Helps to look after the women we deliver from our independent practice, and the role of these Mother's Helps is specifically to mother the mother after she has had her baby. We think that it is very important for women to spend at least 10 days to a fortnight based in their bedroom, just with their new baby. This means that if they have other children they are accessible to the other children, but are quite boring because of being in bed. The other children do not feel that their mother has gone away and they have access to their mother and their mother can read them stories and entertain them, but at the same time is able to rest and get to know the new baby. For a first time mother it is just as important to think through the labour and the huge change in one's life that having a baby brings, and the job description we give to our Mother's Help is as follows:

YOU ARE
THE ICING ON THE CAKE

Welcome to this new family.

The couple you have just met have been through one of the most enormous and life changing experiences of their lives. The woman has been through an arduous physical endurance test and her partner has been through a time requiring great stamina and strength from him. They are both tired and they both need cherishing over the next few days and weeks.

Here's where you come in!

We have advised the new mother to stay in bed for at least 10–14 days to get to know her new baby and to help her to assimilate all that has happened during her labour and her delivery. Your job is to help in this process by virtually mothering the mother (and/or parents).

You are employed to make the 2 weeks after the baby's birth one of the most precious times this couple will ever experience.

The times you work should be negotiated with the new parents, but normally we expect you to work from 9.30 a.m. to 3.30 p.m. or 10.00 a.m. to 4.00 p.m., or other combinations of this.

You should aim to ensure the new mother has one or two periods of sleep each day and you should ensure that she is well fed, has plenty of drinks and feels cherished.

This is a new mother and baby – please increase her self confidence by praising her efforts and by being very complimentary. She does not need you to look after the baby in any way but if she has other children, the children will need to be organised, played with, given meals, etc., etc.

In a nutshell we expect you to be the mother in the household for the period you are here. To provide meals and drinks, do washing and ironing, light housework, to do shopping, prepare an evening meal and to look after the children like a second mother.

A suggested routine for the day is:

1. Make a cup of tea/coffee and breakfast of toast, honey, jam, cereal – neatly laid out on a pretty tray.
2. Run mother's bath for her and while she is in the bath make her bed (changing sheets as necessary).
3. Dust, tidy and hoover throughout home, clean bath, lavatory and washbasins – empty bins.
4. Mid morning coffee (or other drink) for mother (and you).
5. Prepare lunch (omelette, salad, toasted cheese, beans on toast, scrambled egg, etc.).
6. Wash up. Put washing on (or do this earlier in the day so that it is hung up by the time you leave).
7. Go shopping – if there are other children, take them to the park or entertain them with stories while mother has a rest.
8. Prepare supper or vegetables.
9. 3.30 p.m. Leave.

*   *   *   *   *   *   *

This is not an original idea – in Holland such women have been in operation for years, they have a training which enables them to also do postnatal checks on both mother and baby as well as looking after the whole family (van Teijlingen and McCaffrey, 1987).

The other incredibly important 'Health Care Assistants' in my life are Marie and Alison who are my own Mother's Help/Home Help. They do the housework, ironing, clearing up and cleaning in my home and by so doing enable me to work as a midwife. They look after Phil when he comes to mend any doors, or locks or chairs and generally keep this midwife going. All these people, although not called Health Care Assistants, are doing exactly that role.

We need to explore the different jobs that we can delegate to other people. It is ridiculous for midwives to be doing secretarial duties, or cleaning or checking equipment, we need to grow more aware that our time is very precious and expensive, every second counts and should not be frittered away on ironing, peeling potatoes or writing letters which can all be done by other people who don't have a midwifery qualification. Midwives should be doing midwifery.

A reluctance to delegate jobs

Many women find it exceedingly difficult to delegate work that they see as 'their work'. It is as if women have been brought up with the notion that anything to do with domesticity has to be their work and that to ask somebody else to do it for them is idle or a delegation of responsibility. I have had ridiculous arguments with very senior midwives who have blithely told me that they enjoy doing their ironing, my response to them has always been, "you are one of the most senior people in my profession, I want you to be out there fighting for me, my profession and women. Other people could be doing your ironing, only you can lead my profession forward – please don't waste your time".

Why do women have this very punitive attitude to themselves and to 'their' work? Perhaps it has been bred into us since we were little girls that we should be doing all the work in the house, but in our day and age this is hardly fair and equitable, when husbands help women and expect to take their share of the work in the household more and more, can it be right for expensively trained and highly skilled midwives to be doing work that could be done by less expensive personnel?

Health care assistants within the NHS

On reading the preceding paragraphs I can hear you saying to yourself "Oh Pooh to you Caroline Flint, your totally irrelevant description of the assistance you have as a rich independent midwife is something that I really don't want to hear about and is getting up my nose".

I am aware that my practice is obviously outside the NHS and may appear to have no relevance to midwives working within the NHS. The reason that I have listed the assistance and helpers that I personally employ and who we as a practice employ is in order to open our minds to the different ways of helping that different Health Care Assistants can provide. We tend to think of Health Care Assistants as the old 'Nursing Auxiliaries' – whilst these staff members are extremely useful, it might be worth looking at whether assistance of a clerical type might be more useful for midwives, or of a housekeeping type.

In the *Nursing Times* of 19 June 1991, Marie Manthey, describes a primary nursing system in which each patient has one primary nurse who has 24-hour responsibility for him or her. She describes in her unit how each Senior Nurse has an Auxiliary Worker who is 'bonded' to the Senior Nurse, so that every Senior Nurse has a partner who does the same shifts, does the same schedule and has the same holidays and takes care of the same caseload of patients as the Senior Nurse. Thus the two workers, the Nurse and the Auxiliary Worker, always work together and the patient gets to know both of them. The patients are aware that the Auxiliary Worker cannot decide or do such skilled work as the Senior Nurse but the partnership appears to work very well indeed. Manthey describes the advantages of using a partnership approach in that it cuts orientation time in half – this type of working may appeal to you in your work as a midwife, it may enable you to increase your output enormously, on the other hand the type of Health Care Assistant you need may be someone who can help with putting the discharges on the computer, who can write a quick letter to the woman's GP, who can ring the SHO and tell him about baby Brigg's sticky eye – if you are fortunate they may be one and the same person.

Housekeepers

In many areas in the NHS and in GP's Services Housekeepers are being employed. The Housekeeper is there to oversee the general running of the ward or practice and her role is to ensure that stocks are adequate, that there are adequate refreshments for people who cannot get up and get their own refreshments. She generally oversees the comfort and general smooth running of an area.

In some Hospitals the Antenatal Clinic is run by a House-keeper or Health Care Assistant, she has no midwifery skills but she has a lot of skills in making people comfortable and helping the smooth running of the area. In a Labour Ward a House-keeper can make all the difference in the world. Her presence can mean that there is always an amnihook available, that all the cupboards have labels on them so that a visiting midwife can find whatever she is looking for. It means that in every room in the Labour Ward there is written (and available) the Syntocinon regimen for that particular Unit. In an age when even green beans have instructions on the packet on how to cook them, it would seem even more important to have instructions printed in a Labour Ward where there can be a life or death situation. It can take a month or more to learn where everything is kept in a Labour Ward and how 'we do it this way' in a particular Unit. If cupboards, shelves and containers are labelled so that it is easy for a midwife coming in from the community with a woman to see where the intravenous infusions are kept or what exactly women have in this Unit when they have an epidural, then the smooth running of the Unit is enhanced, as is the comfort and safety of the woman having her baby there.

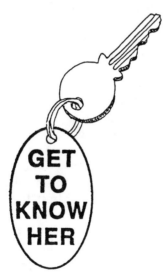

12

Independent midwives in partnership

I have been married to my beloved husband for 29 years, and when times are hard with my business and professional partner – Valerie Taylor – I often say a marriage is much easier and much more simple than a business partnership. When Giles asked me to marry him 30 years ago I just said yes and we proceeded to tell everybody and arrange our wedding. When Val and I decided to go into partnership as midwives it was much more complex.

First, we went to see an accountant, to discuss the way we should be running our accounts, and then he drew up a partnership agreement which bound us both to work with each other and ensured that if either of us was to leave we should have to give 6 months' notice. We agreed to share the profits of the business equally. We then took the partnership agreement to a solicitor who tidied it up and we both signed. We named ourselves 'Special Delivery Midwifery Practice'.

We set up a joint bank account and on the security of both our flats, we obtained a joint overdraft to cover the costs of setting up our business. Finally, we went to a photographic studio and had a photograph of ourselves taken which was to go on the back of our brochure. We had enormous help from women we have delivered in the past or who had been to our antenatal classes. One woman, Helen, drafted our information packs for us and advised us on a reasonably priced printer so that we could get all our literature printed. We needed headed notepaper, envelopes, brochures, information packs, pens, calculators, a photocopier and a telephone answering machine.

Val and I needed to live off our overdraft and we needed to spend it very carefully because it was difficult to see where our clients would come from. We both needed reliable, clean and efficient cars and we looked into leasing arrangements and buying. Val made a very good arrangement with a local garage and she beat them down in the purchase of two cars. In retrospect we realised that we should not have used our overdraft to buy two cars because this left us very short of ready money and our budget became very tight, it probably would have been more sensible to lease our cars, leaving us more money available.

We needed to buy equipment. I had been practising for some time as an independent midwife so only needed a new sonicaid, I already had got the rest of the equipment. We bought bags, Entonox equipment, we arranged a contract with British Oxygen for hiring Entonox cylinders and we arranged an account at the local pharmacy and with one of the big medical suppliers in Wigmore Street. We sat down and worked out the amount it would cost us in equipment, tests, ultrasound scans, sanitary towels, delivery packs, mileage and petrol to deliver a woman. We added a percentage so that we could be paid and we then had our brochures printed and we started to advertise.

In Special Delivery Midwifery Practice we have several objectives: number one is obviously to earn our living in a pleasant way by looking after women and delivering their babies. Two, is to increase choice for women throughout the country, to this end our aim is to increase the home birth rate to 30% by the year 2000 because we feel that if a third of women are having their babies at home, women actually have real choice, whereas when only 1% of women are having their babies at home, only the strongest and the most assertive of women are able to choose to have their babies at home.

In order to change the fashion that nearly all women have their babies in hospital we are attempting to make it 'fashionable' to have a baby at home, therefore we are targetting those women who change opinions and who lead fashion. We are targetting MPs' wives, journalists, actors, wealthy upper middle class women who other women aspire to emulate. This policy is frequently criticised by our friends and colleagues because it is seen as elitist, which it undoubtedly is, but it does seem quite a good way of turning the tide of opinion and the reason that we can do it is because we practise in London, where a great number of the independent midwives provide a marvellous and virtually free service for women who cannot afford to pay.

We started by advertising in such journals as *Harpers and Queen*, and the local National Childbirth Trust newsletters which is cheap to advertise in and reaches a middle class clientele. We placed Nationwide advertisements in the National Childbirth Trust's Baby Annual, and we have always tried to have a number of national advertisements in order to help women to know that they could deliver their baby at home inside the NHS as well as outside it. We also keep the list of all the Independent Midwives in the country handy to help women to contact them who want to – we also have a small network of midwives throughout the country who will deliver women at home who work under our auspices, they have their equipment supplied by us, their blood tests arranged by us, we try and give support and often we write letters on their behalf and advertise locally for them. This has taken off more slowly than we anticipated but we are aware that we have enabled quite a few women to have their babies at home who otherwise would not have been able to.

We frequently put women in touch with Margaret Whyte, of the Society to Support Home Confinements, and with Beverley Beech, at the Association for Improvements in the Maternity Services. Many branches of the National Childbirth Trust now have home birth support groups. All these different organisations help women to achieve greater choice and help women who are contemplating having a home birth to feel supported and normal and not total freaks!

Val and I are very different in character and although our philosophy is the same when it comes to birth – our approach, our outlook and the way that we do things are very different. One of the most important parts of our practice is that we meet each other every week and we sit down to talk through all matters concerning our practice. The other more painful thing we have tried to do is to be totally honest about each other to each other, especially about those things which we are finding aggravating in the other partner. It can be very difficult to hear that somebody you are close to and you respect finds your behaviour unacceptable, distressing to learn that you frighten and overwhelm people. It is painful to tell somebody that you are not happy with the way they conducted a consultation or with certain words they used.

When two people work so closely together they are bound to hurt each other if they are totally honest with each other, but if one contemplates working with a partner for a decade, one needs to get past external appearances and develop a much deeper understanding. It seems to me that this naturally occurs in a marriage and the tussle and struggle between the personalities is in many ways easier than it is in a business partnership. I may just be being subjective because my husband is very easy going, or it may just be that in a marriage the difficult patches are always made easier by the physical relationship, but for both Val and I working in a partnership has at times been hard but it has also brought enormous joy, satisfaction and personal growth for us both.

Having delivered several women who had been left over from my independent practice when working on my own, Val and I then had a launch of Special Delivery Midwifery Practice. One of our aims has always been to publicise the work we do as much as possible, first, to make it more accessible to women and, secondly, because we wanted to act as role models for midwives, and show midwives what they could do and how they can work outside the NHS if that is what they want to do.

We had our launch at the Royal College of Midwives on Thursday 15 November 1990, and several journalists came as well as friends, parents we had delivered, midwifery managers, and relatives. It was great fun and we were very pleased with the caterers Val had organised – the food was marvellous. We gained a great deal of media exposure from our Launch – it made us realise how useful this was and that it was something we must do as regularly as we possibly could!

One of the most important aspects of being self-employed is keeping accounts, and the discipline of accounting for every item of expenditure and every cheque or money coming in. It is essential to do this on a day by day basis because if allowed to mount up it is inordinately difficult to remember what you spent £15.35 on on 14 March or 3 July, but if you do it on the day that you buy the photocopying paper and 36 pens it is easy to remember. We have an account book which has 22 sections and at one end we write down the money we pay out each month, and we keep either the invoice or a copy of the invoice and a copy of the receipt so that they are easily accessible, and at the other end of the book we list the money that comes into the practice. All our clients are regularly invoiced so we are able to put the invoice number next to the payment in.

Valerie and I are both always on call and, except for when we have days off, we answer our bleep according to how close we are to a telephone. We both have car telephones; Val has a telephone in her bedroom and I have my telephone in the room next door to my bedroom, so we invariably have access to one. If the bleep goes off in the night and we need to go out we seem to have evolved a very comfortable way of handling the calls – our biorhythms are very different, late in the evening I am exceedingly tired while Val is just about coming alive, so that if we are called at 9, 10 or 11.00 p.m. at night Val usually goes out, but on the other hand if we are called at 2, 3 or 4.00 a.m. I am wide awake having had a few hours sleep whereas Val is like a zombie, so I go out. We seem to divide the work up fairly equally between ourselves, some days one of us does more than the other, but the other invariably catches up and we pay ourselves an equal amount at the end of every month.

Other practices work in a different way. Some practices pay per antenatal visit, per postnatal visit or per labour, so that the person who has done 25 antenatal visits and 65 postnatal visits and three labours will tot all those up and charge the practice for those, and the person who has done less will get paid less. It is one way of working and is quite useful if one partner is more heavily committed with more children, or more dependants than the other.

We have found our secretary/assistant to be absolutely invaluable. Although we have an answering machine many people are nervous about leaving messages, and if they can actually speak to a human voice they are much more chatty and find it much easier to talk. Janet has learned a great deal about midwifery over the years and is able to answer many questions, especially the question about the way that we practise. She also runs our invoicing system and produces letters for Supervisors of Midwives, GPs and she fixes up appointments with the ultrasound scanning department and generally underpins the partnership by relaying messages to our car telephones and keeping us up to date with what is happening in the office when we are away on visits all day, so that we are prepared for what might be a change in our programme for the day.

In our practice we book four women a month, some months we might book five and some months we only get three or two, but our normal and target number is four. The theory is that we deliver one woman a week and as each woman has about 18 hours' antenatal care, 18 hours' postnatal care and anything up to 20 hours labour care this involves a high degree of commitment of time. Obviously primigravid women normally take longer during labour than multigravid women, but this is not always the case and sometimes with a gravida four, for instance, she is sure she is in labour but there is actually no cervical dilatation, but you are afraid to leave her because if she says that she is in labour she undoubtedly is, and you know that the minute you get halfway down the M4 she will be bleeping you to say that she is pushing, so sometimes we just take up residence in the house and sleep and eat there waiting for the labour to get going.

We do not work out the number of hours that we do but sometimes it feels as if we are working 24 hours a day and other times it is boring because we do not have enough to do. Births tend to come in clusters so that we will have three births in 1 week and we will then have 3 weeks of postnatal visiting and antenatal visiting and getting into a slight panic because we are wondering whether we have forgotten how to deliver a baby. All in all it leads to variety and it is very stimulating working in such a way.

As our clientele increases we intend to take on a third midwife but we intend that women should only get to know two of us because we think that any more than two is probably more than women would want to get to know. It does mean that we will be able to have more regular holidays and that it will not be so stressful for the remaining midwife when somebody goes on holiday. Even with just two of us we still have holidays, although sometimes those holidays are broken into when somebody goes into labour and an instant cancellation of the holiday happens and the holidaying midwife leaps into action – but to be quite honest this is usually because she can't bear to miss someone's birth and the other could have coped perfectly well on her own. If one of us needs to go away for a considerable period, such as over a month, we will employ a locum, but this is costly and very complicated in that the women need to meet the locum before they go into labour and they find it disturbing that they might be delivered by somebody that they do not know very well, and also because we have got so used to working with each other it might be quite hard working with another person. Often, if one of us is away, the other just carries a list of other independent midwives that she can call on if things become very fraught but usually the remaining midwife just gets on and does all the work.

Office work

One of us has taken on the paying of all the bills, which necessitates being in the office for some time every week, otherwise we get behind with paying our bills and we get rude letters from our laboratories or we get our credit card stopped, so regular paying of bills is essential and being freed to do that is a necessity. For our secretary we need to arrange every day those letters that need to be written and they need to be dictated and organised. This involves one of us dictating for 1 or 2 hours every morning and it means getting up very early so this can be carried out. The perks of this are that any letters either of us needs to have typed can be done along with the Special Delivery correspondence and things that need to be chased up during the day, such as the Entonox delivery or getting the next batch of Syntometrine – these can be carried out by Janet on our behalf during the day while we are out on our visits.

Supervisors

Val and I work in London and our clientele live anywhere within the confines of the M25 or just outside it. This means that we actually work in about 26 Health Authorities, and we have to fill in 26 Intention to Practise forms every year and we have to liaise with 26 Supervisors and as most areas have more than one supervisor, often more. Every Supervisor expects an Intention to Practise form filled in from us, she also has the right to inspect our equipment, our notes, our premises and the way we practise.

It is patently impossible to liaise meaningfully with 26 supervisors so we have made an arrangement with most areas that one Supervisor from each Regional Health Authority (and we are dealing with four) will check our equipment, registers and notes each year and will write a letter which we can show to other Supervisors of Midwives that our practice and our equipment are satisfactory.

Another way that we deal with this – and improve relations with Supervisors at the same time – is that we invite all the Supervisors of Midwives to a lunch party, and we do this in April or May each year. We lay out all our equipment, our records, our registers and examples of our notes and we put on a lunch. We have a slide show of women we have delivered and we have a presentation which consists of showing the Supervisors of Midwives our statistics, they are always fascinated by the whole set-up and we enjoy the day getting to know all the different Supervisors.

The role of Supervisor of Midwives is an exceedingly difficult role and one wonders whether it is really absolutely necessary. It is obviously essential that a woman who is being looked after by any professional person should have an avenue for complaint and be assured that that complaint will be dealt with fairly and realistically. Women who are looked after by independent midwives (or indeed by any midwives) have access to the UKCC Investigating Committee to whom they may report any incidences of poor midwifery practice that is meted out to them. The role of the Supervisor of Midwives is unique amongst any professions, no lawyer has a supervisor of lawyers, no doctor has a supervisor of doctors, no architect a supervisor of architects. We are the only profession where a client can be perfectly satisfied with the care that she has received, and in fact so can her GP, her local Obstetricians and anybody else one might care to mention, but the Supervisor of Midwives can intervene, can ask to discuss the notes, and to see the notes and can generally make life unpleasant for the independent midwife with her inquiries even though nobody else has any complaints whatsoever.

Supervisors of Midwives themselves are not always sure of their role in that frequently their experience of home birth is extremely limited and when they are talking to a midwife about a particular incident they often find it difficult to appreciate exactly what was going on at the time and to visualise the whole scenario, often because of lack of experience in practice in that environment.

On the other hand a Supervisor of Midwives who is supportive can be an enormous help and support both to the midwife and to the woman she is looking after. One of the best ways of bringing out the very best in supervision of midwives is to enlist the help and support of the Supervisor on specific matters so that they are able to do something extremely useful for the midwife, who is able to appreciate their help and actions and so improve relationships between them both.

For instance, in our practice we always let the local Supervisor of Midwives know that we have booked a woman in her area for a home birth. In the letter we also go on to say that if we need to transfer our client to hospital we would like to carry on looking after her, so can the Supervisor please assure us that this will be possible. Some of the Supervisors then issue us with an Honorary Contract and others just go on to say of course you can come in to look after Mrs Bloggs, there will be no problem at all.

But in some instances the Supervisor will write back and say I am sorry but it is the policy of our Obstetricians that only those midwives employed inside the Unit can provide midwifery care. This can mean that the Supervisor is very blinkered and is just going along with the Obstetrician – not her role as Supervisor at all, but more often it is the Supervisor having an enormous battle with the Obstetricians who could actually do with a bit of support from midwives from outside the system to help her to open up the Maternity Unit and the minds of the Obstetricians. So we then continue a correspondence about how important it is to the woman that she has continuity of carer especially if she has had to be transferred into hospital whilst anticipating a home birth because she will not only be disappointed at the change of venue, but she will be disappointed in her own body for not working in the way that she hoped it would and she will also be feeling very vulnerable and distressed, therefore it is essential that she is looked after by a midwife she has been able to get to know.

Sometimes we approach one of the Consultants that we know in that Hospital and appeal to his better nature, because he is flattered and interested in our courting of him and frequently we are given permission to take a woman into hospital 'on this occasion only' and this has then opened up the possibility for other midwives to go into the hospital and look after their clients. If this doesn't work the next port of call is the local MP – whilst at the same time making sure that we have a friendly hospital to take the woman to in the case of needing to. It also shows the Supervisor of Midwives and the Obstetricians that women's wishes must be respected. As well it underlines that independent midwives are responsible practitioners and do not bring harm or disrepute to their Unit, but actually quite the reverse.

Sometimes we ring a Supervisor of Midwives because we are feeling isolated and somewhat concerned, for instance at the time a woman had a twelve hour second stage but was not willing to be transferred into hospital. We rang up a Supervisor of Midwives to discuss how we should proceed and to get some professional support and this was most generously given.

First of all the Supervisor ascertained that the fetal heart and the mother's condition were satisfactory, which they were. Then the Supervisor suggested that we should try and negotiate a time limit with the woman so that if the second stage went on for very much longer we would actually have a time when we knew we could transfer her to hospital. The Supervisor also suggested that having used a pinard's stethoscope all the way through the labour because our client did not wish us to use a sonicaid, we should try and insist on using a sonicaid so that we could all hear the fetal heart more easily, we managed to negotiate with our client that we could use a sonicaid but she was not willing to discuss a time limit because she thought that that would put her under pressure. The reassurance and support from that Supervisor certainly changed our feelings of anxiety to one of security, in that we had professional support, and that there was somebody thinking about us and aware of how things were progressing.

In the end the baby delivered beautifully, and it was quite obvious from later discussion with the Supervisor that the baby's position had been persistent occipitoposterior and that infrequent uterine contractions during the second stage of labour had put very little pressure on the baby's head and enabled the baby to withstand quite comfortably a long second stage of labour with no distress at all – the baby was finally delivered at home in very good condition and continues to thrive.

There have been occasions when we have run out of our ample supplies of Entonox and we have telephoned the local Supervisor of Midwives and said HELP! to her and she has sent a Community Midwife around with two or three cylinders of Entonox which we have then replaced the following week. In some areas Supervisors of Midwives will lend independent midwives equipment or will arrange blood testing through the hospital for them. Many Supervisors value discussions with independent midwives because it gives them ideas for their own midwives' practice and we notice how much the Supervisors enjoy going through our bags and our equipment and jotting down items of equipment that they had not seen before and are thinking of buying for their staff.

Another example of superb support from a Supervisor was following the delivery of a small baby born at 37 weeks. The baby became jaundiced on day 2 and we needed to take a serum bilirubin, we took the serum bilirubin – rang the Supervisor from the car telephone as we approached the hospital. Her secretary was at the entrance to meet us, escort us to SCBU for the relevant forms and chart, then to the pathology laboratory where we made arrangements for them to bleep us with the result. We were only in the hospital for 10 minutes and the whole thing was organised like clockwork – so useful when time is precious.

One of the main aspects of working outside the NHS is the need to maintain good relationships with all those health professionals who the midwives are likely to come into contact with. We always keep the woman's GP very well informed about the progress of her pregnancy and the results of blood tests and ultrasound scan. We write a letter to the GP immediately the woman has booked us and in the letter we assume that the GP will not wish to be involved in intrapartum care or postnatal care but we invite the GP to come and examine the baby within the first few days of its life. We need to make it quite clear in the letter that we are taking full responsibility for the woman's maternity care, otherwise GPs have the notion that all health issues are their responsibility and because it is very rare for a GP to be involved in intrapartum care we need to make it clear that we do not expect him/her to be involved and we are quite happy doing it on our own. In the same letter we point out that if we have any problems or complications we will contact the local Maternity Unit and transfer the woman there.

We have twice received angry letters from GPs who have been offended by the assumptions we have made that they will not wish to be involved in the woman's care during pregnancy, labour or the puerperium, but usually when we explain to them that in 2 years we have only had three replies to these letters and most GPs do not even acknowledge the letters we send to them, they soon understand why we need to write in the way that we do. We always have problems in liaising with the Health Visitors because in every area they seem to be based in a different place and attached to somewhere different, but as the Health Visitor usually arrives on Day 11 and we go on regularly visiting until Day 28 we can normally liaise through our client and we suggest to our client that she shows the Health Visitor the notes of her labour and birth so she obtains the full picture.

We have several hand-picked Consultant Obstetricians who each have specific and very useful skills. When our clients go over 42 weeks of pregnancy we have excellent relationships with a fetal assessment unit to which to refer our clients, so dealing with two issues at a single stroke. First, by ensuring that the pregnancy is progressing well and, secondly, enabling us to comply with Rule 40 of the Midwives Rules, "in any case . . . where she detects in the health of a mother and baby a deviation from the norm a practising midwife shall call to her assistance a registered medical practitioner", because the woman automatically sees a Consultant Obstetrician when she goes to the fetal assessment unit that we use.

Sometimes we refer to an Obstetrician at his rooms in Harley Street who is very good at turning breeches, although we would dearly love to develop this skill for ourselves. If we need to refer a woman to hospital we always hand pick the Consultant Obstetrician we are going to refer to, because we want to work with those Obstetricians whose philosophy and aims and approach are similar to our own. Usually, if we respect them and the way that they practise they also respect us and the way that we practise, and our relationships are usually very pleasant and also very productive because we learn a lot from each other.

One Professor of Obstetrics keeps us very up to date with the latest research on many aspects of maternity care, and his advice and good counsel is invaluable.

It is also important to have good relationships with your suppliers and to this end we have an equipment book in which we name all our contacts in those places we order goods from and we have the identification number of the specific sanitary towels, inco pads or Syntometrine that we order. This means that we can keep a record of when we order goods, when we received them and when we paid for them, and when we need to re-order, we can do this very quickly.

Obtaining supplies

We have an account with a local chemist and with one of the big medical suppliers in Wigmore Street, and this is very useful because it means that we can order those medications and equipment that we need very quickly and we are charged by invoice at the end of each month.

For blood tests and ultrasound scans we use a private laboratory and a private ultrasound facility. Both of them invoice us at the end of each month. For those who work within the NHS, with blood tests being lost and results taking a long time to be returned, let me describe to you how it can be.

First of all you order from the laboratory all the facilities you need for taking blood – these are vacutainers, needles, needle holder, padded envelope, stamped addressed labels and forms. When you have taken the blood, or collected the urine, or performed the swab, you put it inside the padded envelope with the form, which only needs the woman's name on it and a description of the test you require (most of these are ordered by just ticking a list of tests available), it is then put inside the padded envelope, the label is put on to the envelope and the whole thing is put into the nearest post box. Within 3 days the results arrive by post.

Our practice has three printouts of results, one for us, one to send to the GP and one for the woman's notes. If we needed four sets of printouts we would be sent four sets of printouts, if we needed only one we would be sent one, because this is a private laboratory and it is catering to each individual customer and each individual customer's needs are taken note of. If there is an abnormality such as the haemoglobin level being very low, or an infection in the urine, the laboratory rings us and informs us immediately so that we do not have to wait for the results to come by post before we take action.

The printout not only has the results of the woman's blood, or urine, etc., it also has the range of normal values and those values which are abnormal in the specimen are highlighted. Does this service cost a fortune? No. Does this service ever fail? Not to my knowledge and I have been using it for the past 12 years. In an emergency, at weekends, or at Bank Holidays, there is always a haematologist or bacteriologist on call and they can deal with the specimen immediately. Before now, when I have taken the blood from a rhesus negative mother and dropped it into the laboratory on a Sunday morning the result has been at my home before I have got there and the journey has only taken 20 minutes. This is how easy blood tests can be for the person taking the blood, with the results coming through quickly and with a printout which shows the practitioner when an abnormality is occurring – no hassle, no problems, just information. It is wonderful!

Our equipment has to be up to date as does our knowledge of relevant research, recently we have had to do literature searches on the effects of vitamin K, dehiscence of scar following a previous caesarean section, the effects of epidural anaesthesia and breech births and their mortality rates. Women who are employing their own midwives expect a high standard of knowledge and information – it keeps us up to date and interested, it is a most stimulating way of working.

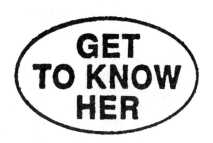

13

Staffing a Birth Centre or GP Unit

GP Unit staffing

Our plan is that Special Delivery Birth Centre will open in September 1993. When you read this book it may be up and running, on the other hand we may be still struggling in our attempts to set it up. The idea is that women, who would normally be perfectly eligible to have their baby at home, have been so frightened by the prevailing philosophy in obstetrics and by all the adverse media cover about having a baby at home that they are too afraid to go all the way and have their baby at home.

Our intention is to set up several Birth Centres, preferably in the perimeter road of a hospital or in a house outside a hospital, so that we have ready access to an operating theatre for caesarean section or other interventions. Instead of the woman having her baby in her home, the woman will come and have her baby in our home, but the fundamental intention will be that this is a home and not an institution and the basic principle is as ever that she will have somebody with her who she has been able to get to know during her pregnancy.

The intention is to have rooms that look like normal sitting rooms with a sofa in them and carpet on the floor and with a birth tub in the corner so that women can use that if they want to. We also plan to have an en suite lavatory and shower off each bedroom. Our reasoning is that we are able to deliver women very comfortably in their own homes and we do not leave behind any stains or mess anywhere, so there is no reason why we should not be able to do that in our own home.

As the Birth Centre is a home the front door will be closed until somebody knocks at it and it is opened by somebody on the inside.

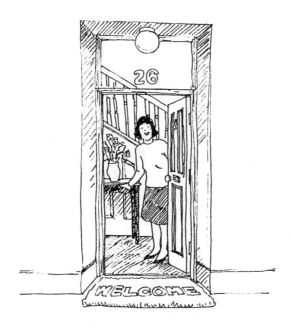

People will not be able to walk in and out of our Birth Centre. All women in labour inside the Birth Centre will be as assured of privacy as they are in their own home. In the kitchen will be all the things you find in your own home: eggs, bread, butter, jam, Marmite, fish fingers, baked beans, milk, tea, coffee, orange squash, orange juice, apple juice, salads, bacon, fruit, cheese, marmalade and biscuits. The people staying in our home will be able to come and make themselves snacks or we will make snacks for them. There will be televisions, radios, comfortable sofas.

One of our aims is that there will be a gradual realisation within the whole NHS that there is absolutely no need for women to labour and give birth in rooms which are so disfunctional for this purpose. Women in labour need surfaces to lean on, they need a soft floor on which to crawl and kneel, they need comfortable chairs and an ability to move, lean and recline. It is virtually impossible in most Labour Wards for them to be able to do this, there is no need for the wards to look as they do at the moment, they could look just like your bedroom or my sitting room. If the birth centres become popular there will be a growing realisation of that fact and labour wards throughout the country should change, we hope they do.

Staffing of the Birth Centre

How will the Birth Centre be staffed? In a word – it won't. The women, however, will be staffed and the woman will have a midwife who she has been able to get to know during her pregnancy and who will have her own caseload.

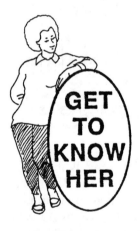

In our Birth Centre we are planning to pilot the scheme which we think would be appropriate for midwives working within the NHS – every midwife taking on a caseload of 36 women, and this is exactly how we will run the Birth Centre. We shall employ one midwife at the beginning and that one midwife will take on 36 women during the first year. Once we get to booking more than 36 women we will employ a second midwife and from then on they will book 36 women a year each and will liaise between themselves as to when they are going to take their holidays and when they are going to cover for each other. This will free up both the midwives and they will be able to arrange their lives around their work and their social life.

Both the midwives (and eventually all the midwives) will carry long range bleepers and they themselves will liaise with the women they are going to deliver in the Birth Centre. They will do all the women's antenatal care in the Birth Centre where we shall have two consulting rooms, and they will also provide the woman's labour, delivery and postnatal care in the Birth Centre until she leaves and goes to her own home. If the woman is within a reasonable distance of the Birth Centre the midwife will carry on her postnatal care at home, but if she lives a very long way away the midwife will liaise with the local Community Midwives for postnatal care, but the midwife will still keep in touch with the woman by telephone and will arrange for the woman and her baby to come to the Birth Centre from time to time to be seen by her.

The Birth Centre will need ancillary staff. It is likely that we shall employ a domestic/housekeeper to clean the house, launder the sheets, order supplies in the house and also to cook meals for those women who are staying in the house at the time and for those midwives who are working in the house at the time.

We may need an administrator/secretary as well, or this role and the housekeeper role may be combined in one person, this is yet to be decided.

GP Unit/Midwife Led Unit staffing

There are many GP/Midwife Units in the country. These Units have been providing maternity care for women in their locality for many, many years. They provide a friendly, low tech, non-invasive form of maternity care and are popular in their areas but invariably they suffer from too few women using them.

Whenever I visit one of these GP/Midwife Units I get excited at the thought that I am going to be seeing beautiful normal midwifery carried out in a normal and friendly setting, and always I am bitterly disappointed and I can absolutely understand why women do not take advantage of these units.

Why? I suggest that the reason why women do not avail themselves of GP/Midwife Units is because they are invariably set up as mini hospitals and the birthing rooms look exactly like a delivery room in the most high tech of hospitals, there is invariably a narrow, high, hard, delivery bed on which the woman is supposed to labour and deliver. There is invariably a plastic crib against the wall, a resuscitaire and a fetal monitor. There may be a chair for the 'husband', the floor is as hard and inhospitable as the floor in any high-tech maternity unit. There are still no surfaces for the woman to lean against, no soft bags or sofa for her to flop against.

If we know that up until the early sixties 90% of women in this country had their babies at home, what on earth are we doing trying to persuade women to have babies in places that look more like operating theatres than somewhere where women give birth? One of the most refreshing sets of recommendations in the Health Committee Second Report on the Maternity Services (The Winterton Report) is paragraph 327 and 328 which state:

> It is clear that many women find it beneficial to be free to adopt whatever position feels right during labour and birth and a growing number find birthing pools helpful in labour and/or delivery. We recommend that all hospitals make it their policy to make full provision whenever possible for women to choose the position which they prefer for labour and birth with the option of a birthing pool where this is practicable.

and

> The environment in which a woman gives birth is very important. If the home setting is considered as the model on which to base care, a hospital delivery unit should:
> — afford privacy
> — look like a normal room rather than be reminiscent of an operating theatre
> — enable refreshments to be available for the woman and her partner or companions
> — ensure the feasibility of the woman being "in control" of her labour. All case notes should contain the woman's wishes for her labour

— enable the woman to take up those positions in which she is most comfortable

— enable the woman to have with her a midwife she has been able to form a relationship with during her pregnancy.

The other disadvantage that many GP/Midwife Units suffer from is the continuation of the shift system as if this was again a high-tech Maternity Unit. Invariably the midwives are staffing a place instead of staffing women, either the Antenatal Clinic, the Postnatal Ward or the Labour Ward, the midwives in many GP Units staff the whole Unit but still this means that they are staffing the Unit rather than staffing the women.

In GP/Midwife Units midwives often say that the women know them all because there are so few midwives working in the Unit and often they have been there for such a long time. This may be true of women who have had several babies in that Unit, but for women having their first baby there seems to be very little attempt to enable women to have their own midwife or pair of midwives. One only has to think of Pithivier, the Unit run by Dr Michel Odent, a few kilometres from Paris, which was a small Unit available to women in the locality, but women trekked from all parts of France and from the United Kingdom and other countries to that small Unit in order to give birth there. Surely, there is no reason why many of the GP/Midwife Units could not be in exactly the same position, with women making a pilgrimage to them from all over the country. Invariably this does not happen because women do not know about them and because they are still not offering women what women ask for, which is to be enabled to form a relationship antenatally with the midwife who is going to be with them in labour.

Midwives' caseloads

If the midwives in a GP Unit decided to staff women rather than the Unit they would be with the woman whenever and wherever she needed them. This is 1993 and we have advanced electronic communication. Midwives anywhere in the Western World have access to bleepers and message pagers and the use of telephones, they can always be contacted. Therefore if each midwife working in a GP Unit takes on a specific caseload of women and works as described earlier and works in partnership with another midwife, between them they can take on at least 72 women a year and can provide all their antenatal, labour and delivery and postnatal care.

During the postnatal period if the woman stays in hospital they may need to use a Health Care Assistant who provides hotel-like care; if the woman is at home during this period a Health Care Assistant in the form of a mother's help or home help is extremely valuable. Midwives who take on their own caseloads in this way would find an enormous boost in their self-confidence and would be able to practise fully as midwives. The women in their care would appreciate being looked after by the same two midwives throughout their pregnancy, labour, delivery and the postnatal period, and the service could be ideal. I suspect that if any GP/Midwife Unit set up such an ideal way of providing continuity of carer and publicised it they would find that women would flock from all over the country to have care with them, because this is what women have been asking for for so long.

Postnatal care

Many women will choose to leave the Birth Centre soon after the baby has been born, some will want to stay on for longer. Who will look after them during this postnatal period, who will care for them? Again we shall model the running of our Birth Centre on the type of care that women who have babies at home receive. Women who have babies at home are looked after for most of the day by their husband, their mother, the next door neighbour, their friend or an employed mother's help (shall we call her/him a Health Care Assistant?).

There is always controversy as to who should be providing postnatal care and it is important that the woman should have almost instant access to a midwife in case she bleeds or has a problem with her baby. Perhaps the time has come to look at every woman having her own midwife and having access to that midwife in a crisis so that the midwife can direct operations over the phone and can hurry to the woman's side. This concept makes many people feel insecure but for those women w would otherwise have been able to have their babies at home is there any reason why this type of care should not be the norm for these low-risk women?

Obviously women who have had a caesarean section, who have actually had surgery and need real nursing are in a different category from those women who have had a normal birth, no episiotomy, may be just a few stitches and who have not lost a great deal of blood and who are tired and stiff but otherwise healthy.

In Chapter 7 I have reproduced rotas from a Birth Centre in Sydney, Australia, there they do not have their own caseloads, they work shifts and they rely on the women getting to know them because there are so few midwives working in the Birth Centre. I hope we see a growth of Birth Centres in this country, places which look homely and are comfortable, where women can labour and deliver with the minimum of obstetric intervention. So far we are not seeing any great increase in such places, and those which do operate often have an extraordinarily long exclusion list – no primigravidae (who needs gentle and sensitive midwifery care more than anyone else? This experience is going to colour the rest of this woman's life and certainly her subsequent pregnancies and labours), no women who have not been tested for HIV (I am not making this up – it really happens), no one who has had a previous caesarean section, no woman who is over 35, no woman having a fourth baby – I can go on and on. If we try hard enough the definition of normal can be squeezed down to a woman (preferably white), over 5 foot 6 inches, with black or blond hair (never ginger!), whose feet are size 6 and above, who has had either one or two previous children weighing at least 8 pounds and who is aged between 25 and 31. Please read this list and recognise that so much of it is nonsense and based on no research evidence whatsoever.

14

Conclusion

I hope this book will help you to set up a continuity of carer scheme for the women you have the privilege and delight of providing care for. It is essential that we provide continuity of carer for women, we cannot go on ignoring their pleas any longer. It is never easy to initiate change and all change is exceedingly hard to live through, but having achieved radical change in the way described it would appear to me that many benefits will come about, not just for women, but also for midwifery as a profession.

As the Presidents of The Royal College of Obstetricians and Gynaecologists, The Royal College of Midwives and the Chairman of Council of The Royal College of General Practitioners said in their joint paper in 1992:

Maternity care forms the very basis of good health. The outcome of pregnancy can affect the future physical and emotional health of the individual woman and the potential of her baby to achieve optimum health. Good maternity care is health promotion at its most positive.

The three Presidents go on to describe a framework for maternity care in the future:

Women do not need to be "sold" any one type of care – the majority are in control of their own lives and are used to making decisions. In pregnancy this capacity is enhanced by a strong desire to maintain health and to promote the health of the unborn child. Clear and unbiased information about the options for antenatal care and the place of delivery should be provided wherever a woman makes first contact with the health service. The woman's own views and preferences should be a very significant factor in formulating any programme of care. It has to be recognised that these may not always coincide with the opinions of her professional adviser.

How exciting that our three Colleges have recognised that it is women who should have the deciding vote in the type of care that they should be receiving. It is women who need to be in control of the whole process because after all they are going to be in control of this child until he or she becomes an adult. Ann Oakley (1980) showed in her study 'Transition to motherhood', that women who feel in control of the situation when they are pregnant and in labour are less prone to postnatal depression. The other week I listened to an American woman in her late seventies, describing in intimate and very exact detail the birth of her son which took place nearly 50 years ago. Her clarity of memory of that, so significant, event in her life was as clear as if the birth had happened last week. We need to remember that for women the memories surrounding their first birth experience never leave them. They are part of that woman for the rest of her life.

It appears to me that those people who will have the most effect on the maternity services have to be those people who provide a continuum of care throughout the whole experience, through pregnancy, labour, delivery and the puerperium. Midwives are in the strongest position to effect change and to provide a more responsive service for women. Consultants stay in a hospital for many years, but this is not true of registrars or indeed of housemen. GPs provide a continuum of care throughout a person's life but most GPs provide antenatal care and often one-off postnatal care, there are very few (very dedicated and very much appreciated) GPs who actually provide intrapartum care.

The people who are there for years and who have experience of and who provide the whole continuum of care are midwives. As the three Presidents said in their statement:

> Midwives have the most experience of pregnancy and childbirth as a normal event and they are the responsible professional at the majority of births. Midwives provide antenatal care including parenthood education, intrapartum care and care of mother and baby in the postnatal period. They work in the community in collaboration with general practitioners and in hospital in collaboration with obstetricians and this flexibility enables them to provide continuity of care within pregnancy. As midwives provided the bulk of practical clinical care in pregnancy and childbirth it is important if women are to experience a continuity and convenient care that midwifery services are organised

appropriately. Thus, it is the view of the Colleges that midwives require identifiable caseloads.

The Presidents of the three Colleges acknowledge the importance and necessary input from those women who have been receivers of maternity care:

> Local Maternity Service Liaison Committees or similar groups provide General Practitioners, Midwives, Obstetricians and lay people with an essential forum. Through these they are able to establish practice guidelines based as far as possible on research to ensure consistency of care and to enhance and to clarify professional relationships. Fully functional Liaison Groups with equal professional membership and with lay representation should exist in all health authorities.

This is a call for women from the consumer groups to be listened to. One of the most revealing and humbling factors for me in my recent experience as an adviser to the Select Committee on the Maternity Services was that I realised for the first time in my professional life I was experiencing an astonishing phenomenon – for the first time in my life I was aware that women were being listened to. Ordinary women, women who had just had babies, women who were experts in the whole process of the Maternity Services because they had just been through that experience. I hope that we can take that example further and that I shall again during my professional life experience the phenomenon of women being listened to.

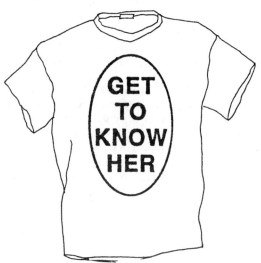

It is time that we listened to women and it is time that we heeded the huge amount of research that has been done into childbirth. We need to look at the way we give advice to women and to try to maintain an unemotional view of the advice we give, and to give the woman all sides of the question and also to give her the most up to date research information that is available to us. It is no longer acceptable for any of our profession to say 'this is what I would do'. As Iain Chalmers was quoted as saying in *The Independent on Sunday* on 13 September 1992, none of us should be guilty of "A failure to recognise that opinions unsupported by strong evidence cannot be expected today to be as influential as they have been in the past in shaping maternity practices". Women are well educated and they are the people who pay for the services that we provide whether that is within or without the NHS. It is our duty to give them all the information that we have available to us.

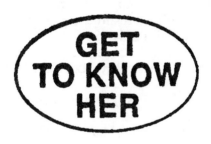

References

Allison J. (1992) Midwives step out of the shadows. *Midwives Chronicle* **105**, (1, 254), 167–174.

Association of Radical Midwives (1986) *'The Vision' – Proposals for the Future of the Maternity Services*. ARM, 62 Greetby Hill, Ormskirk, Lancs L39 2DT.

Ball J. (1992) *Birthrate. Using Clinical Indicators to Assess Case Mix, Workload Outcomes and Staffing Needs in Intrapartum Care and for Predicting Postnatal Beds Needs*. Cost £11.50p from The Nuffield Institute for Health Service Studies, 71–75 Clarendon Road, Leeds LS2 9PL.

Biro M. and Lumley J. (1991) The safety of team midwifery: the first decade of the Monash Birth Centre. *Medical Journal of Australia* **155**, 478–480.

Boyd C. and Sellers L. (1982) *The British Way of Birth*. Pan Books, London.

Buchan J. and Stock J. (1990) *Midwives' Careers and Grading*. A Report for the Royal College of Midwives. IMS Report No. 201. Institute of Manpower Studies. Mantell Building, University of Sussex, Brighton BN1 9RF.

Campbell R. and Macfarlane A. (1987) *Where to be Born? The Debate and the Evidence*. National Perinatal Epidemiology Unit, Radcliffe Infirmary, Oxford.

Chalmers I., Enkin M. and Keirse M.J.N.C. (1989) *Effective Care in Pregnancy and Childbirth*, 2 vols. Oxford University Press, Oxford.

Chamberlain G. and Zander L. (eds) (1992) *Pregnancy Care in the 1990s*. Parthenon, Carnforth, Lancs.

Cronk M. and Flint C. (1989) *Community Midwifery, A Practical Guide*. Heinemann Medical, Oxford.

Downes E. (1989) Motherhood – team efforts to ease pain of childbirth. *Sunday Times* 23 October (New Society section).

Enkin M., Keirse M.J.N.C. and Chalmers I. (1989) *A Guide to*

Effective Care in Pregnancy and Childbirth. Oxford University Press, Oxford.

Evans F.B. (1987) *The Newcastle Community Midwifery Care Project: An Evaluation Report.* Newcastle Health Authority, Community Health Unit, Newcastle General Hospital.

Flint C. and Poulengeris P. (1987) *The 'Know Your Midwife' Report.* From 49 Peckarmans Wood, London SE26 6RZ.

Freely M. (1991) Assembly-line health services economies that fail to deliver. *Independent on Sunday* 29 September, p. 34.

Haire D. (1981) Improving the outcome of pregnancy through increased utilization of midwives. *Journal of Nurse-Midwifery* **26**, 5–8.

Hale C. (1986) Measuring job satisfaction. Occasional Paper. *Nursing Times* 26 March.

Hall L.W. (1991) Six elements for implementing and managing change. *Leadership and Organization Development Journal* **12**, (2), 24–26.

Hall M.H., Chung P.K. and MacGillivray I. (1980) Is routine antenatal care worthwhile? *Lancet* **ii**, 78–80.

HMSO (1980) *Second Report from the Social Services Committee. Session (1979–80), Perinatal and Neonatal Mortality.* HMSO, London.

Harris C.A. (1989) *Midwife Teams in Riverside Health Authority.* Riverside Health Authority, Finance Department, London.

Heseltine A. and Watkins D. (1991) Team labour. *Nursing Times* **87**, (29), (Midwifery), 40–42.

House of Commons. Session 1991–92. *The Health Committee, Second Report: Maternity Services,* vol. 1. HMSO, London, March 1992.

Houston G. (1984) *The Red Book of Groups and How to Lead Them Better.* The Rochester Foundation, 8 Rochester Terrace, London NW1.

Jacobson B., Eklund G., Hamberger L., Linnarsson D., Sedvall G. and Valverius M. (1987) Perinatal origin of adult self-destructive behavior. *Acta Psychiatrica Scandinavica* **76**, 364–371.

Kennell J.H., Jerauld R., Wolfe H., Chesler D., Kreger N.C., McAlpine W., Steffa M. and Klaus M.H. (1974) Maternal behaviour one year after early and extended post-partum contact. *Developmental Medicine and Child Neurology* **16**, 172–179.

Kidlington Midwifery Scheme (1990) *Report of the Kidlington*

Midwifery Scheme. Institute of Nursing, Radcliffe Infirmary, Oxford.

Kitzinger S. (1981) *Change in Antenatal Care. A Report of a Working Party Set Up For the National Childbirth Trust.* NCT, London.

Klein M., Lloyd I., Redman C., Bull M. and Turnbull A.C. (1983a) A comparison of low-risk pregnant women booked for delivery in two systems of care: shared care (consultant) and integrated general practice unit. I. Obstetrical procedures and neonatal outcome. *British Journal of Obstetrics and Gynaecology* 90, 118–122.

Klein M., Lloyd I., Redman C., Bull M. and Turnbull A.C. (1983b) A comparison of low-risk pregnant women booked for delivery in two systems of care: shared care (consultant) and integrated general practice unit. II. Labour and delivery management and neonatal outcome. *British Journal of Obstetrics and Gynaecology* 90, 123–128.

Klein R. (1983) Mothering instincts. *Health Service Journal* 1 September, p.1057.

Kowalski K., Gottschalk J., Greer B., Watson A. and Bowes J.R. (1977) Ideas and actions. Team nursing. *Journal of Obstetrics and Gynaecology* 50, 116–119.

Macfarlane A. and Mugford M. (1984) *Birth Counts. Statistics of Pregnancy and Childbirth (Tables).* National Perinatal Epidemiology Unit (in collaboration with Office of Population Censuses and Surveys), vol. I. HMSO, London.

Macfarlane A. and Mugford M. (1984) *Birth Counts. Statistics of Pregnancy and Childbirth (Tables).* National Perinatal Epidemiology Unit (in collaboration with Office of Population Censuses and Surveys), vol. II. HMSO, London.

Manthey M. (1991) President of Creative Nursing Management, Minneapolis, USA in her article in *Nursing Times* 87, (25).

Maternity Services Advisory Committee (1982) *Maternity Care in Action. Part 1 – Antenatal Care.* HMSO, London.

Melia R.J., Morgan M., Wolfe C.D.A. and Swan A.V. (1991) Consumers' views of the maternity services: implications for change and quality assurance. *Journal of Public Health Medicine* 13, 120–126.

Menzies I.E.P. (1970) *The Functioning of Social Systems as a Defence Against Anxiety.* The Tavistock Institute of Human

Relations, London.

Metcalf C.A. (1987) Job satisfaction and organisational change in a maternity hospital. *International Journal of Nursing Studies* **23**, 285–298.

Micklethwaite Lady P., Beard R. and Shaw K. (1978). Expectations of a pregnant woman in relation to her treatment. *British Medical Journal* **2**, 188–191.

Neil C. (1985) *Delivering the goods*. Nursing Times, 30 January, p.19.

Nuffield Institute for Health Service Studies (1992) *Who's Left Holding the Baby? An Organisational Framework for Making the Most of the Maternity Services*. £7.50 from The Nuffield Institute for Health Service Studies, 71–75 Clarendon Road, Leeds LS2 9PL.

Oakley A. (1980) *Women Confined*. Martin Robertson, Oxford.

Oakley A., Rajan L. and Grant A. (1990) Social support and pregnancy outcome. *British Journal of Obstetrics and Gynaecology* **97**, 155–162.

Ong B.N. (1983) *Our Motherhood*. Family Service Units, 207 Old Marylebone Road, London NW1 5QP.

Parents (1983) Birth in Britain. A *Parents* special report. A survey of 7500 women's views. *Parents* 92.

Parents (1986) BIRTH 9000 mothers speak out. Birth survey 1986 – results. *Parents* 128.

The Patient's Charter Group (1992) *The Named Midwife*. Gratis from Patient's Charter Group, Room 758, State House, High Holborn, London WC1R 4SX.

Pearse I.H. (1979) *The Quality of Life, The Peckham Approach to Human Ethology*. Scottish Academic Press, Edinburgh.

Pearse I.H. and Crocker L.H. (1943) *The Peckham Experiment – A Study of the Living Structure of Society*. Scottish Academic Press, Edinburgh.

Plant R. (1987) *Managing Change and Making it Stick*. Fontana, London.

Robinson S. and Thomson A.M. (1991) *Midwives Research and Childbirth*, vol. II. Chapman and Hall, London.

Royal College of Midwives (1991) *Towards a Healthy Nation. Every Day a Birthday*. The Royal College of Midwives, London.

Royal College of Obstetricians and Gynaecologists (1982)

Report of the RCOG Working Party on Antenatal and Intrapartum Care. Royal College of Obstetricians and Gynaecologists, London.

Royal College of Obstetricians and Gynaecologists, The Royal College of Midwives and The Royal College of General Practitioners. (1992) *A Framework for Maternity Care. Maternity Care in the New NHS – A Joint Approach.* Royal College of Obstetricians and Gynaecologists, London.

Runnerstrom L. (1969) The effectiveness of nurse-midwifery in a supervised hospital environment. *Bulletin of American College of Nurse-Midwives* **14**, 40–52.

Slome C., Wetherbee H., Daly M., Christensen K., Meglen M. and Thiede H. (1976) Effectiveness of certified nurse-midwives. *American Journal of Obstetrics and Gynecology* **124**, 177–182.

Stein A. (1986) Breech delivery, a co-operative nurse-midwifery medical management approach. *Journal of Nurse-Midwifery* **31**, 93–97.

Stirrat G.M. (1988) Chapter 5. In: James D.K. and Stirrat G.M. (eds), *Pregnancy and Risk – The Basis for Rational Management.* John Wiley, Chichester.

Sunday Times (1987) *LIFEPLAN.* William Collins, London.

Tew M. (1990) *Safer Childbirth? A Critical History of Maternity Care.* Chapman and Hall, London.

van Teijlingen E. and McCaffrey P. (1987) The profession of midwife in the Netherlands. *Midwifery* **3**, (4), 178–186.

Welsh Office NHS Directorate: Welsh Health Planning Forum (1991) *August 1991 Maternal and Early Child Health. Protocol for Investment in Health Gain.*

Which (1989) Your baby, your choice. In: *Which? Way to Health.* Consumers Association, London, p.13.

Wright C. (1989) The domino effect. *Nursing Times* **85**, (15), 37–38.

Index